# BENEFITS OF PLANT BASED MEDICINE

*A patients guide to plant-based medicine, essential oils and natural remedies that can treat, heal and prevent disease*

**Howard Mason**

# © Copyright 2019 - All rights reserved.

The content contained within this book may not be reproduced, duplicated or transmitted without direct written permission from the author or the publisher.

Under no circumstances will any blame or legal responsibility be held against the publisher, or author, for any damages, reparation, or monetary loss due to the information contained within this book, either directly or indirectly.

Legal Notice:

This book is copyright protected. It is only for personal use. You cannot amend, distribute, sell, use, quote or paraphrase any part, or the content within this book, without the consent of the author or publisher.

Disclaimer Notice:

Please note the information contained within this document is for educational and entertainment purposes only. All effort has been executed to present accurate, up to date, reliable, complete information. No warranties of any kind are declared or implied. Readers acknowledge that the author is not engaging in the rendering of legal, financial, medical or professional advice. The content within this book has been derived from various sources. Please consult a licensed professional before attempting any techniques outlined in this book.

By reading this document, the reader agrees that under no circumstances is the author responsible for any losses, direct or indirect, that are incurred as a result of the use of information contained within this document, including, but not limited to, errors, omissions, or inaccuracies.

# Table Of Contents

**Introduction ........................................................... 6**
   The Side Effects of Prescription Drugs Are Silent
   Killers ................................................................................. 7
   Do Plant-Based Medicines Really Work? ........................ 9
   What You Will Learn in This Book ................................. 10

**Chapter 1: The Early Days of Medicine ................... 12**
   Herbal Medicine and Ancient Egyptians ....................... 13
   The Effectiveness of Ancient Egyptian Herbal Medicine .. 15
   Ancient Egyptian Herbal Healing Was Adopted by the
   Rest of the World ............................................................. 17

**Chapter 2: The Evolution of Medicine .................... 20**
   The History of Pharmaceuticals ..................................... 20
   The History of the FDA's Role in Modern Medicine ......... 25
   Herbal Medicine is the Enemy of the Pharmaceutical
   Industry ........................................................................... 29

**Chapter 3: Choosing Your Doctor - Why it
Matters ................................................................... 31**
   The Difference in a DO vs. MD Doctor ........................... 31
   What a Typical First-Time Visit to a DO Doctor is Like ... 32
   The History of Osteopathic Medicine ............................. 33
   Treating Symptoms vs. Preventing Illness ..................... 33
   The Doctor's Internal Interest in Prescribing
   Pharmaceutical Drugs .................................................... 37
   How to Choose the Right DO Doctor for You ................. 38

**Chapter 4: The Holistic Approach .......................... 41**
   The Holistic Doctors' Strategy ........................................ 42
   Herbal Remedies and Holistic Healing .......................... 44
   Why Insurance Companies Will Not Cover Holistic
   Treatment ........................................................................ 48

**Chapter 5: Your Immune System** ......................... **50**
   What is the Immune System?............................................. 50
   The Parts of the Immune System ..................................... 51
   Disorders of the Immune System......................................53
   How Processed Foods and Pharmaceutical Drugs Can Negatively Affect the Immune System .............................53
   How to Maintain a Healthy Immune System....................55
   Plant-Based Foods That Help to Boost the Function of the Immune System............................................................57

**Chapter 6: Cleanse and Rejuvenate Your Body** ..... **60**
   What is a Detox?................................................................. 60
   Reasons Why You Need to Detox ....................................... 61
   How Does Detoxing Work? ................................................. 62
   Benefits of Detoxing .......................................................... 62
   Common Ways of Detoxing................................................ 63
   Additional Ways to Help Your Body Detox.......................73

**Chapter 7: Plant-Based Diet** ........................................**76**
   What are Processed Foods?................................................76
   What is a Plant-Based Diet? ..............................................81
   Benefits to Practicing a Plant-Based Diet ....................... 85
   How to Transition to a Plant-Based Diet ........................ 86
   7-Day Plant-Based Meal Plan............................................ 88

**Chapter 8: Essentials Oils** ........................................**91**
   What are Essential Oils?.....................................................91
   The History of Essential Oil Use ....................................... 92
   What is Aromatherapy?...................................................... 93
   How Essential Oils Work.................................................... 94
   Other Uses of Essential Oils .............................................. 95
   Types of Essential Oils and the Part of the Plant That They Are Derived From ..................................................... 95
   Popular Essential Oils and Their Health Benefits........... 99
   The Dangers of Improper Usage of Essential oils .......... 100
   The Do's and Don'ts of Using Essential Oil Safely ..........102

**Chapter 9: Herbal Medicine .............................. 104**
What are Medicinal Plants? ............................................104
Probiotics ....................................................................... 115
List of Herbal Remedies .................................................. 118
**Chapter 10: Medicinal Garden ............................123**
Benefits of Planting Your Own Medicinal Garden .......... 123
Planning Your Garden ..................................................... 125
9 Common Herbs and Spices That You Can Grow on
Your Own ........................................................................128
**Conclusion ........................................................ 137**
Plant-Based Medicine Worked for Our Ancestors and It
Can Work for You Too .................................................... 138
Plant-Based Eating Can Change Your Life for the Better 138
Take Control of Your Overall Health ............................... 138
**References ........................................................ 141**

# Introduction

Just as plants provide us with powerful nutrition, they also provide us with powerful medicine that can treat anything from the common cold and influenza right down to cardiovascular disease, diabetes, and cancer. Headaches, diarrhea, malaria, asthma, pneumonia and tuberculosis are also common health issues that can be treated with herbal sources, and they only constitute a small portion of the long list.

Herbal or plant-based medicine is not a new concept. In fact, plants have been used medicinally for thousands of years. From the leaves and stem down to the bark and roots, plants were used to not only treat diseases, illnesses and abnormalities but also as a source of prevention.

If plants are so effective in treating so many common health issues, why are synthetic medicines being pushed down our throats, both literally and figuratively? The answer is both simple and appalling. Treating illnesses has become a big business. Pharmaceutical companies thrive on human illness and on providing temporary solutions in the form of prescription drugs. Synthetic medicines most often do not treat the root of an illness and as such the symptoms do not truly go away. The symptoms are only masked and typically recur.

Most pharmaceutical products contain ingredients derived from plants. The list of these includes aspirin, opium, quinine, and digitalis. Pharmaceutical companies have learned to capitalize on the active compounds in plants to replicate their effects temporarily.

Nothing beats what nature has provided. More than 80% of the population of developing countries depend on plants to treat medical ailments while more than 60% of the entire global population does the same. This is so not simply because plants are a cheap source of powerful relief. So many people count on herbal medicines to heal their bodies and completely change their lives because they are also accessible and plentiful. Almost anyone can plant a garden and grow common medicinal plants. In fact, many of the plants that we will discuss in this book are household names. They include chamomile, garlic, gingko, peppermint, ginger, and ginseng.

Despite the effectiveness, great availability and affordability of herbal medicine, drugs provided by pharmaceuticals are still considered a superior source of medicine by many even with the many side effects that they generate and how ineffective they often are.

## The Side Effects of Prescription Drugs Are Silent Killers

Side effects can range from mild to life-threatening. In using these prescription drugs to cure one medical problem, we often have to deal with unexpected medical problems that these drugs manifest within us.

Common 'mild' side effects that are related to the use of prescription drugs include:

- Headaches
- Dry mouth
- Diarrhea
- Dizziness
- Dermatitis or skin rashes
- Constipations
- Nausea

- Insomnia
- A general feeling of being unwell

While these are labeled as mild by pharmaceuticals and some doctors, I would say that the inconvenience and the pain they cause are far from minor. These effects disrupt daily living and can lead to more serious medical issues.

Some of the more serious side effects that can occur with the use of prescription drugs include:

- Internal bleeding
- Heart disease
- Increased blood pressure
- Liver damage
- Cancer
- Mental issues like depression and anxiety disorder, which can lead to suicidal thoughts and actions

No one knows how their bodies will react before taking a prescription drug, and the risk, which is your life, is too great to put on the line. The side effects of taking prescription drugs cannot be reversed. The sufferer has to deal with the consequences for the rest of their life, and the solution that pharmaceutical companies and some doctors offer is even more prescription drugs that can induce even more side effects. This is a vicious cycle that has to stop.

Discontinuing prescription drugs can also have negative effects on the user. Some of these drugs can cause dependency and addiction, and thus, the user will experience withdrawal symptoms after discontinued use. Withdrawal symptoms can cause sweating, shaking, nervousness, nausea, bone pain, sleep issues, depression and more.

## Do Plant-Based Medicines Really Work?

Although almost 40% of Americans have admitted to using herbal medicine to attain excellent results, there is still much skepticism toward the effectiveness of plant-based medicine. This is because plant-based medicine and supplements are not required to be FDA approved before they are made available to the public. The FDA (Food and Drug Administration) does not regulate herbal medicine because it is considered a dietary supplement rather than a drug.

However, there have been many RCTS (randomized controlled trials) that have provided evidence to support the legitimacy of the effectiveness of plant-based medicine. These tests have isolated many active compounds of several plants to show their health-related effectiveness.

One of these compounds is called capsaicin. It is the active compound in chili peppers that induces the burning sensation in the mouth when consumed. Despite what may be an unsettling sensation to some people, this compound has a long history of effectiveness in treating pain, such as low back pain, osteoarthritis, peripheral diabetic neuropathy, and postherpetic neuralgia. Qutenza is an FDA approved substance that uses chemically synthesized capsaicin to imitate the same effects.

The active compound in butterbur, a plant that is a member of the daisy family, has been shown to be a remedy for fighting pain, wounds, ulcers and inflammation. Ancient Greeks used it because of its powerful effects. It has also been synthesized to be used in migraine medications.

Green tea is another common herbal remedy. It is made so effective by its high concentration of polyphenols. Polyphenols are plant compounds that help boost brain health and improve digestion. They can be used to treat dementia, coronary artery disease, cancer, and diabetes. Their effects are so widespread that a 2015 systematic review concluded that increasing tea consumption of any kind reduces the risk of developing cardiovascular diseases such as stroke and cardiac death.

The active ingredients menthol and methyl salicylic are found in peppermint, which is a hybrid between water mint and spearmint. These active ingredients help treat a number of ailments, including irritable bowel syndrome, skin irritation, migraine headaches, tension headaches and non-ulcer dyspepsia. A 2014 study stated that peppermint oil was more effective in fighting the symptoms of irritable bowel syndrome, such as bloating, gas, diarrhea and pain, compared to a placebo. Another study in 2016 found that peppermint oil reduces the frequency and intensity of irritable bowel syndrome symptoms.

The list of evidence to support the effectiveness of plant-based medicine goes on and on.

# What You Will Learn in This Book

This book is jam-packed with insight and knowledge such as:

- The history of pharmaceuticals and how they have convinced us to live with the side effects of prescription drugs
- The history of plant-based medicines
- How to choose a doctor who truly has your best interest at heart
- How to implement a holistic approach to attacking the root of your illness instead of just treating symptoms
- How to detox your body from harmful toxins
- The benefits of detoxing

- How to implement a natural wellness plan to improve your overall health
- How to incorporate a plant-based diet in your life
- How to maintain a medicinal garden even if you have limited garden space
- So much more!

This book was written to show the harmful side effects that prescription drugs have on not only on your body and mind but on your entire life as well. It was also written to show that there is a healthier alternative that is all-natural, abundant, and cheap. That alternative is a plant-based approach to medicine and eating. My promise to you is that you will gain incredible value from every page that you read in this book. My hope is that you will use this newfound knowledge to inspire you to take a proactive approach to improve your health and wellness by the time you read the last page.

You only get one body and one life. You need to do what it takes to ensure that you treat your body with the utmost love and care. It is time to stop damaging it with the toxins left behind by prescription drugs and the consumption of processed and unhealthy foods. It is time to stop dealing with the adverse side effects gained from something that was supposed to help you and not introduce a new set of problems in your life. It is time you take a plant-based approach to not only medicine but your diet and general living. You owe it to yourself to treat your body right, and there is no better way to treat yourself than with what nature provides free of charge.

Turn the page and discover a whole new whole to illness prevention, treatment, and cures.

# Chapter 1: The Early Days of Medicine

The ancient Egyptian culture was a civilization that lasted from 3300 to 525 BCE. The ancient Egyptians felt that spiritual and physical health were intertwined and so they went to great lengths to ensure that physical health was maintained. The ancient Egyptians believed their gods created and controlled life through magic, demons, evil spirits, and other mythical entities. For example, some people called on the god, Serket, to heal a scorpion bite. It was thought that bad luck, disasters, and physical maladies were caused by angering the gods and dealing with evil forces. Therefore, it was not uncommon to use magic and religion to treat people. It was probably during that civilization that the concept of health began as some of the earliest records of medicine came from that period and civilization.

The healers of those times prescribed both prayer and natural remedies to patients to solve their medical problems. It is for this reason that priests were considered medical professionals. Also, there were two other types of medical practitioners, and they were magicians and healers. Magicians executed spells and charms to get rid of evil spirits that were thought to cause physical maladies. The healers were also called 'swnw.' They employed medications to cure physical ailments.

Although ancient Egyptians had limited knowledge of anatomy, they reached a level of understanding and discovery that allowed them to know that the heart pumps blood through arteries and veins to provide the body with blood. They were also aware that liver infection could cause disease even though they did not know what the specific causes were. This insight and more came from the practice of preserving deceased bodies as mummies so that the human body could be studied.

Despite the knowledge they had obtained, they were also false conceptions like a woman's uterus floated within her body and that vaginal discharge needed to be treated. Despite these false assumptions, ancient Egyptian medical practices were highly advanced for the time and included simple noninvasive surgery procedures, the setting of bones and dentistry. Their practices were so advanced that they influenced later traditions like the Greeks. In fact, by 500BC, Egyptian medicine had become so revered and respected that Egyptian healers were invited by the rulers of Rome and Babylon to visit their courts. Aspiring healers from Greece and Rome went to Egypt to become knowledgeable about these practices.

## Herbal Medicine and Ancient Egyptians

Ancient Egyptian medicine was not just about ideologies on gods and magic but also resulted from experimentation and observation. Much of this experimentation was facilitated by the mummification process, which allowed the extraction of internal organs such as the brain, lungs, liver, spleen, heart and intestines. Along with this knowledge of anatomy came the familiarization of drug preparation as plants and herbs, as aloe, cumin, fennel, castor oil, and pomegranates were used to treat illnesses and diseases. This represented the start of natural medicine. Modern scientists can study this evolution of herbal medicine from a few still-existing papyri, which are journals that were used to document the medical advances of that time.

For example, the Ebers Papyrus on ophthalmology, diseases of the digestive system, the head, the skin and specific maladies, a compilation of earlier works that contains a large number of prescriptions and recipes states that plans medicines includes cannabis, opium, henna, thyme, cassia, juniper, and linseed oil in addition to the few mentioned above. Many of these herbal remedies were soaked in wine so that they could be taken orally. This document listed 876 remedies that were made from over 500 plants.

Here are just a few of the plants ancient Egyptians used and the maladies they fought:

- Garlic. This was given to patients who suffered from bronchial and asthmatic conditions. It was also used to aid in endurance. Garlic was mashed with olive oil. This was ingested to fight the common cold. Fresh, raw garlic was also wrapped in cheesecloth or muslin and then attached to the underwear to prevent the flu and the common cold.

- Onion. This was also given to aid endurance in addition to aiding digestion.

- Cloves. They were mashed and mixed with water and vinegar to form a mixture that was gargled to treat sore throats and toothaches.

- Cumin. The seeds were considered a stimulant and were used to prevent flatulence.

- Coriander was used to treat digestive issues, as a cooling agent and as a stimulant. Both the seeds and plant were cooked in dishes to prevent flatulence. The leaves were brewed to make tea to prevent urinary tract issues like cystitis.

Medical prescriptions were written by the healers to dispense this aid. The prescription typically began with a description of the medication and was followed by ingredients and measures to be used. The method of preparation and how the final product was to be taken, whether it be as an ointment, inhaled, or by other means was included as well. This was a very sophisticated system.

## The Effectiveness of Ancient Egyptian Herbal Medicine

It is true that the ancient Egyptian medical healers did not always get it right. While injuries would be easier for them to understand and treat, diseases were a bit more difficult. This is because injuries were a clear cause-and-effect type of treatment while the causes of diseases were not always clear and so diagnosing was problematic. Therefore, ancient Egyptians thought that the cause of disease was a consequence of displeasing the gods, that the patient was under demonic attack or that the person was being haunted by a ghost. Therefore, disease was treated through the recitation of magical spells rather than with physical methods.

During the ceremony, ancient Egyptian magicians used amulets, aromas, incantations, tattoos, and more to try to drive away demons and gods and to placate the gods so that the disease could be removed. Needless to say, this was not very effective in curing or preventing popular diseases such as malaria, smallpox, pneumonia, cancer, heart disease, dementia, arthritis, high blood pressure, tuberculosis, appendicitis, kidney stones, liver disease and ovarian cysts, all of which were diseases that were common in that time.

Circumcision was a process that was also often met with failure as temple priests performed it using a flint blade as they recited incantations on boys between the ages of 10 years and 14 years. Circumcision was done to mark the boys' transition from adolescence to manhood. Unfortunately, most times this procedure resulted in infection. Since the cause of the infection was unknown to the Egyptians, it was considered the result of the influence of gods, demons and ghosts and dealt with by using magical spells. This resulted in the death of a lot of young men.

Another area that ancient Egyptians had difficulty treating was eye problems. These problems were dealt with by giving the patient a dose of bat's blood because it was thought that the ability of night vision would be transferred to the patient. Ancient Egyptian rulers also failed when dealing with female issues. Fumigation of the womb was most commonly prescribed and followed by incantations because it was believed that the womb was connected to all the parts of a woman's body. Again, this was less than effective because the cause of the problem was not treated; therefore, it persisted.

Fortunately, there were many areas that ancient Egyptians got it right apart from the use of herbal medicine to treat injuries. Healers underwent medical training to learn the profession in a school that was called the Houses of Life. This training consisted mostly of reading texts created by earlier famous healers but there did include some practical study as well.

Ancient Egyptian methods of diagnosis were so advanced that some of them are still being used today. In addition, ancient Egyptian doctors adopted an ethical code centuries before the Hippocratic Oath. The Hippocratic Oath was an inscription that stated, "Never did I do evil onto any person." Ancient Egyptian healers approached medicine in a way that kept the needs and safety of the patient as the first priority.

Dentistry was also an area that ancient Egyptians excelled. They were well aware of how to drain an abscess, how to extract teeth, and even how to make false teeth.

Ancient Egyptian healers were also knowledgeable about how to suture a word. This was done by placing raw meat upon the wound to facilitate healing and stimulate blood production. Honey was also used because ancient Egyptians were aware of its antiseptic qualities and ability to activate the presence of white blood cells, which are the chief component of the immune system. The immune system is the body's defense force against infection from dangerous invading cells such as bacteria and viruses. Even before the discovery of penicillin, ancient Egyptians healers used moldy bread as an antibiotic.

Ancient Egyptian medicine outdated both Roman and Greek medicine in both its level of knowledge and sophistication. This undoubtedly could have been attributed to the practice of embalming the dead during the mummification process. This allowed the ancient Egyptian healers to study the structure of the body and facilitated learning what parts of the body were responsible for certain tasks. Despite the limitations of the equipment and knowledge in that time, ancient Egyptians were excellent physicians. Without the results of their research and experimentation, a lot of the procedures and practices in modern medicine that have saved millions of lives would not have been possible.

## Ancient Egyptian Herbal Healing Was Adopted by the Rest of the World

The famous Greek physician called Hippocrates (450-380BC) became familiar with the herbal medicine practices of ancient Egyptians. He used this knowledge to describe 256 healing herbs. He also developed precise instructions for herb collecting and the categorization of foods and herbs by four basic qualities, which were hot, cold, damp and dry. He then theorized that disease was caused by an imbalance of the four liquids in the body of blood, yellow bile, black bile and phlegm. He stated that good health depended on keeping these in balance because they had great influence over the body and emotions.

These theories on the use of herbal medicine continued to move west and by 100 BC, the theories developed by Greek medicine had reached Rome. Around AD70, a Roman army physician called Pedanius Dioscorides described 600 medicinal herbs in his five-volume publication called De Materia Medica. This publication outlined when leaves, stems, roots, and flowers should be collected as well as when herbal remedies should be prepared. This publication had an enormous influence on medicinal practices for more than 1500 years. This influence was so significant that this was one of the first books printed after the invention of the printing press.

Around the same time, a Roman author, philosopher, and naturalist called Pliny the Elder offered a comprehensive guide that cataloged an extensive list of herbs, which were valuable as medicines. This catalog went on to become an invaluable reference for the Greek physician and philosopher called Galen (AD 130-200). Galen was the court physician to the Roman emperor Marcus Aurelius. He developed the first classification system that paired common illnesses with herbal remedies. His writings went on to become the standard for physicians of the time while the writings of Dioscorides became the standard for pharmacist of that time.

Even though the Roman Empire fell in the 5th Century, the teachings of herbal medicine moved east to Persia and Constantinople. This movement encouraged the merging of folk medicine and Egyptian traditions.

The practice of using herbal medicines continued to spread around the globe and became adopted by many more different cultures such as Arab culture, Latin culture, and through out to Europe.

Due to the invention of the Guttenberg printing press in 1440, herbal medicine writings became more popular. One such publication was written by John Gerald and was called *The*

*Herball or General History of Plants*. This was published in 1597 and was very popular because it was written in English, which meant that there was no need for knowledge of ancient languages for it to be understood.

By the turn of the 17th Century, John Parkinson published the groundbreaking works called Paradisi in Sole Paradisus Terrestris and Theatrum Botanicum, which highlighted more than 3000 plants. He was the first writer to attempt botanical classification by dividing the plants into families and classes. Many more botanists, herbalists, physicians, and astrologists went on to print works that expanded on this knowledge.

Unfortunately, it was also around the 17th Century that there was a decline in the use of herbal medicine and a shift toward the use of pharmaceutical drugs. By the 19th Century, the demand for specific drugs surged, and it seemed that many of the herbal teachings of the past were lost.

# Chapter 2:
# The Evolution of Medicine

## The History of Pharmaceuticals

Pharmaceuticals is a multi-billion-dollar industry. In fact, in the year 2017, this industry generated more than 900 billion dollars in profits and it is projected to be worth more than 1000 billion dollars by the year 2021. It is hard to believe that such a huge industry started way back in the mid-nineteenth century and gained its roots in herbal medicine.

Pharmaceuticals actually had its start by sublime traditional remedies that were big based on folk knowledge. These remedies were sold by apothecaries, who are people who prepared and soul drugs and medicines, and pharmacies. Medicine moved from the use of herbal remedies to what it is today because of the scientific revolution, which started in the 17th Century. The scientific revolution took place in Europe near the end of the Renaissance period and continued into the late 18th Century. This revolution marked the emergence of modern science and the development of subjects, such as physics, biology, astronomy, chemistry and mathematics. The advancements made at that time involved a lot of experimentation and changed the way that society viewed nature. The scientific revolution contributed Isaac Newton's 1687 Principia, the "grand synthesis" and the development of the laws of motion and universal gravitation.

The ideas of rationalism and experimentation was coupled with the idea of benefiting from human health, and this gave birth to the pharmaceutical industry as we know it today.

One of the earliest companies to move in that direction was called Merck. The German company was founded in 1668 but transitioned toward a scientific approach to medicine in 1827. The start was made by manufacturing and selling alkaloids. Alkaloids are a class of nitrogenous-based poisons and drugs. One of the most famous of them is called morphine, which is a drug that is typically prescribed to treat moderate to extreme pain. This drug works by targeting signals in the brain to change how the body feels and responds to pain.

Another early starter of the pharmaceutical industry was called GlaxoSmithKline. The company's origin was traced back to 1715, but it only started producing patented medicine in the year 1842. This company started the world's first factory for producing medicine-only products in 1859. The company's first pharmaceutical product was vitamin D, and this was released in 1924.

America was not far behind in joining the pharmaceutical revolution. In 1849, two German immigrants founded Pfizer. The founders were called Charles Pfizer and Charles Erhart. Both men were in their twenties when they started the company in Brooklyn, New York. The first product the company released was an anti-parasitic drug. While sales were moderately successful, it did not put this company on the map. That came in 1862.

Business was slow to start but rapidly expanded during the American Civil War due to the extremely high demand for antiseptics and painkillers. The company catered to demand and doubled its revenue at the start of the war.

Another huge pharmaceutical company called R&D was set up in 1876. This was founded by a former Cavalry Commander in the Union War called Colonel Eli Lilly. He was a trained pharmaceutical chemist and made a move into the pharmaceutical business after the end of his military career.

Lilly was not the only military man to get into the drug business. Edward Robinson Squibb (1819-1900) was a naval doctor during the Mexican-American war that lasted from 1846 to 1848. He used to throw drugs overboard because of the low quality, and in 1858, he set up his own laboratory. He founded the company called E. R. Squibb and Sons, which went on to become part of the modern pharmaceutical super-company called Bristol-Myers Squibb.

Other countries were not far behind to skyrocket the development of the pharmaceutical industry. Switzerland came on board in the second half of the 19th Century. The venture started with a lot of controversies because of the lack of patent laws, which led to the countries being accused of being a "pirate state." Pharmaceuticals in Switzerland started when they realize that the dyestuff they produced had antiseptic and other medicinal properties. They began to market these as medicinal products. This practice showed a clear breach of ethics because there was no differentiation between medicine and other chemicals.

Bayer was another company that initially got its roots in the dye trade. The company made the move to develop pharmaceuticals and commercialized aspirin use at the beginning of the 20th Century. It was one of the most successful pharmaceutical companies of that era. The company was so successful that it had the aspirin trademarked. At the same time, Merck bridged into the American market. In that period, pharmaceuticals were not regulated and the companies took advantage.

Insulin was made available to the market between 1918 and 1939 when Frederick Banting and his colleagues managed to isolate it. This was used to treat diabetes, which was a fatal disease until that time. The first person to benefit from the use of insulin was a 14-year-old boy named Leonard Thompson, who was dying from diabetes. The drug saved his life, and as a result, the news of insulin's effects of diabetes patients spread like wildfire. This led to Banting receiving a Nobel Prize in Medicine.

In 1928, Alexander Fleming discovered penicillin mold's antibiotic properties. Penicillin was the first modern antibiotic developed. This marked a new era for the pharmaceutical industry and its pursuit to develop drugs.

After World War II, the pharmaceutical industry gained more structure, was more regularized, and pricing schemes were introduced. The portfolio of medicinal products grew, but so did the potential ethical conflicts that arose from making money from selling healthcare products.

This lack of ethics was brought into the spotlight in 1961 with the Thalidomide scandal. This drug was marketed as a mild sleep aid and was deemed safe for even pregnant women to use. This drug caused the death of thousands of babies worldwide as it caused the development of malformed limbs.

Thalidomide was developed in the 1950s by a West German company called Chemie Grünenthal GmbH to expand its product range beyond antibiotics. The drug made users feel relaxed and sleepy, and so it was seen as the perfect alternative to tranquilizers, which were fashionable at the time. The drug was patented after testing revealed that it was nearly impossible for an overdose to occur. The testing before this patenting did not include the possible effects during pregnancy. This seemingly harmless drug was licensed in 1956 and became available without the need for a prescription in over-the-counter sales in Germany and almost all European countries. The drug helped ease the symptoms of morning sickness and so sales from pregnant women skyrocketed.

By 1960, the signs that this drug was detrimental to health started to arise. It was found that some users had nerve damage to their limbs after long-term use, and the link between the increased number of babies born with birth defects and the parent's use of the drug during pregnancy was made.

It was estimated that the death toll was over 2,000 children, and more than 10,000 children were born with serious birth defects due to the use of this drug. When taken by a pregnant mother, this drug interfered with the normal development of the baby that the mother carried within.

This scandal prompted an increase in the regulation and testing of drugs before they would be licensed for sale. In the US, there was a new amendment made to the FDA (Food and Drug Administration) rules that demanded proof of efficacy and accurate disclosure of side effects before new medications were released to the market. The Declaration of Helsinki was implemented in 1964 to put a greater ethical structure in place on clinical research so that prescribed medicines had more differentiation from other chemicals.

Since that time, many more drugs have been introduced into the market, such as the contraceptive pill, Valium, antidepressants and antipsychotics. Unfortunately, no matter the great strides made in this industry, side effects have been commonplace from the beginning, and there is no denying that these huge companies benefit from human illness.

This lack of ethics can be seen in the fact that thalidomide was still used after the huge scandal in an effort to treat leprosy, which is a chronic disease that affects the nerves, skin and mucous membranes. Signs and symptoms of leprosy include discoloration and lumps on the skin. Many patients of this disease suffer from deformities and disfigurements. This disease is caused by slow-growing bacteria and is mostly isolated to undeveloped countries such as many African countries.

This drug was placed in use in developing countries to also treat certain cancers and AIDS-related conditions even though its use still remains controversial. The risk of babies being born with thalidomide-related defects has not decreased, so this begs the question of why this drug is still being circulated for use. The answer is simple and appalling—money is being made by the pharmaceutical companies that manufacture them and the corrupt government officials in the pockets of these companies.

## The History of the FDA's Role in Modern Medicine

FDA stands for Food and Drug Administration. The US-based organization has been around for almost two centuries. The role of the FDA is to regulate about one trillion dollars' worth of products every year so that the American consumer remains safe. One of the most famous accomplishments of the FDA was its rejection of the circulation of thalidomide. The company that manufactured the drug sought approval from the FDA to sell the drug in the US in 1960, but this was rejected or when the then FDA inspector Frances Kelsey requested that the company conduct more safety studies. This move placed the FDA in a positive support light and even earned Kelsey praise from the then-US President John Kennedy. The thalidomide scandal helped pass amendments that help strengthen the FDA's drug review process.

Let's go back to where it all started in 1820 when 11 doctors set up the US Pharmacopeia to record the list of standard drugs. This was named the Food, Drug. and Insecticide Administration. This was later shortened to the Food and Drug

Administration in 1930 under an agricultural appropriations act.

It was not until 1848 that the Drug Importation Act was passed by the US Congress to require the customer service to inspect low quality drugs received from overseas. In the following years, companies were required to show proof that the drug that they provided did indeed treat the illness that they claimed.

It was not until 1906 that the original Food and Drug Act was passed by Congress. This was done on June 30th and was signed by President Theodore Roosevelt. This act outlawed States from selling and buying food, drinks, and drugs that have been tainted or mislabeled. This act allowed the FDA to get its first true victory after many decades of fighting for the government to regulate the selling and distribution of food.

The Industrial Revolution occurred in the latter half of the 18th Century and transformed rural societies of Europe and America into industrialized urban areas. It was also called the First Industrial Revolution, and the transition included moving from manual production methods to machines, chemical manufacturing and iron production. This also included the rise of mechanized factory systems and the use of steam and water power.

The Industrial Revolution introduced many consumer demands, and the opportunity for the production of food and medicine rose. As a result, both of these became large-scale enterprises. The shelf life of food was extended with the invention of canning. This allowed food to be shipped farther and to sit on shelves longer without expiring.

On the other hand, patented medicines started being sold to treat a variety of ailments. As we have seen with the medicinal industry, there was a lack of ethics that placed the consumer at a high risk. This was even true for the sale of food and drink products. There were many instances where manufacturers of food and drinks use spices and additives to mask the taste of expired meat and many other substandard ingredients. Manufacturers of patented drugs used cocaine and morphine to give consumers a high rather than actually curing their ailment. Government intervention was needed to protect consumers from this ambiguity and clear lack of ethics. This was a long and hard struggle because manufacturers had a huge influence on Congress through aggressive lobbying.

Luckily, one of the most powerful advocates for the regulation of food and drugs, Harvey Wiley, made huge strides in seeing his dream of making America medicine and food safe for the consumer a reality. He became the chief chemist at the Bureau of Chemistry in 1883 and rallied support to have the Food And Drug Act passed in 1906. His influence was so significant that the law was nicknamed the Wiley Act. He was also given regulation and power of the Bureau of Chemistry so that later amendments and laws were passed.

Unfortunately, there was a hole in this Act as it was found that it did not outlaw false medical claims but only prohibited false and misleading statements about the ingredients of a drug. This was fixed with the passing of the Sherley Amendment in 1912, which outlawed labeling medicines with fake medical claims meant to trick the consumer.

Still, the FDA recommended a total rewrite of the outdated 1906 act in 1933. The need for this rewrite was made apparent in 1957, when an inappropriately prepared medicine caused mass poisoning in the United States. This drug was called elixir sulfanilamide, and it caused the deaths of 107 people. Many of these people were children. The deaths highlighted the need to establish drug safety protocols before drugs were marketed and distributed to consumers.

This led to the passing of the Federal Food Drug and Cosmetic Act in 1938. This act required that a company prove that new drugs were safe for consumption before they were released for sale. This also led to the start of the requirement for prescription-only drugs.

Unfortunately, this was not enough to stop the death of persons at the hands of drug companies. Almost 300 people died or were injured as a result of the use of an antibiotic that was tainted with a sedative in 1941. The FDA changed manufacturing and quality protocols in response to this. This also led to the development of GMP, which stands for Good Manufacturing Practice. This is a system that ensures goods that are manufactured consistently be controlled according to quality standards to minimize the risk of pharmaceutical production that cannot be eliminated through the testing of the final product.

Again, pharmaceutical companies came under fire when an FDA nationwide investigation revealed that an antibiotic caused almost 200 deaths. This led to the FDA engaging the American Society of Hospital Pharmacies, the American Society of Medical Record Libraries, and the American Medical Association to give voluntarily reports of patient drug reactions.

Since that time, many more acts and laws have been passed that give the FDA more power to oversee consumer safety. This is enhanced by growing technology and computer usage. However, the power of the FDA is limited, and even it can't stop the ambiguity of big-name pharmaceutical companies.

# Herbal Medicine is the Enemy of the Pharmaceutical Industry

Naturally healing cannot be patented by big pharmaceutical companies. Pharmaceutical companies will not make money if you simply go out into your garden and pluck up the cure or prevention of a disease. The sad truth is that pharmaceutical companies make big bucks off of illness; therefore, it wants the global society to be sick. There would hardly be a need for prescription drugs if most people were strong, fit, and healthy.

Of the seven billion people on earth, only a small percentage are considered part of the ruling elite. This percentage controls the majority of the wealth on this planet, and of that percentage, the owners of pharmaceutical corporations have a huge seat at the table. Between the years of 2003 and 2012, the top 11 pharmaceutical companies generated almost one trillion dollars in profits.

There has been a shift away from the use of herbal medicine since the development of the pharmaceutical industry back in the 17th Century. Since that time, herbal medications have been suppressed for the use of modern medicine. Healthcare has become a big business, and its rise is dependent on human sickness. Pharmaceutical companies have a big interest in ensuring that we as a global society do not gain information or knowledge on just how effective traditional herbal medicines can be. They also have a vested interest in causing side effects that lead to the further need of drugs that they produce.

One of the most prescribed drugs are painkillers. Painkillers are highly addictive and are not only the instrumental to physical health but mental health as well. Did you know that more than 75% of the US population over 50 years of age is currently taking prescribed medication? Did you know that 25% of women in their forties and fifties have been prescribed antidepressants? Did you know that even though the US population accounts for only 5% of the global population, it consumes more than half of all prescribed drugs?

These are high figures, and they were deliberately calculated and manipulated in existence by big pharmaceutical companies. The use of prescription drugs is an epidemic that is facilitated by an army of doctors. The pharmaceutical companies control was is taught in medical schools, and your doctor may even be unknowingly playing in their hands with your health on the line. The pharmaceutical industry is a system that is rigged to keep humans chronically unhealthy in exchange for dollars.

# Chapter 3:
# Choosing Your Doctor - Why it Matters

## The Difference in a DO vs. MD Doctor

An MD doctor is one who practices allopathic medicine. Allopathic medicine refers to science-based, modern medicine. As a result, this type of doctor will regularly prescribes medication manufactured by pharmaceutical companies to treat illnesses and diseases.

On the other hand, a DO doctor is one who practices osteopathic medicine. Osteopathic medicine refers to patient treatment in a more holistic approach rather than the treatment of symptoms. This is a whole-person approach to medicine.

DO doctors are fully licensed to practice medicine and only differ in their approach to patient treatment. Both types of doctors are licensed to see patients, prescribe medication, and perform surgeries. Therefore, going to a DO doctor does not mean that a patient is compromising their healthcare

The osteopathic approach to medicine that emphasizes that the body's part all work together and influence the function of each other. This is a synergistic relationship that needs to be kept in balance. DO doctors have special training that allows them to perform osteopathic manipulative treatment (OMT). This is a group of hands-on treatment techniques that allows these types of physicians to diagnose, treat and prevent patient illness and injury. As part of a DO's education, there includes special training on the musculoskeletal system. The DO uses this knowledge to move a patient's muscles and joints using osteopathic manipulative treatment techniques that include stretching, gentle pressure, and resistance.

The benefits of OMT are numerous and can help people of all different backgrounds and ages. This treatment can be used to promote healing, increase overall mobility, and ease pain. It has been shown to be of particular benefit to people who suffer from carpal tunnel syndrome, migraines, menstrual pain, asthma, and sinus disorders.

## What a Typical First-Time Visit to a DO Doctor is Like

This includes four parts and they are:

### *The interview*

This is where a patient discusses his or her medical history with the DO doctor. Often, the patient is asked to share information about his or her work, family, and home life.

### *The exam*

The DO will perform a complete medical exam, which includes checking posture, muscles, joints, ligaments, and tendons. Tests like blood work and urine analysis will be ordered if they are necessary.

### *The diagnosis*

This is the part where the DO will consider the results of the interview and exam with input from the patient to determine what is causing the symptoms of whatever ailment it has brought the patient to the DO.

### Treatment

The DO will suggest a treatment plan that is best for the patient and may include osteopathic manipulative treatment. Whatever course of treatment that the doctor prescribes is done to encourage the body's natural penchant toward self-healing.

## The History of Osteopathic Medicine

This approach to medicine was developed by Dr. Andrew Taylor Still in 1874. Dr. Still was inspired to develop this approach to medicine when allopathic medicine failed to save his children from dying of meningitis.

Dr. Still compared the function of the human body to a machine. He reasoned that a machine only functions at optimum when it is mechanically sound and the human body works in the same way. He believed that it is a doctor's role to improve the mechanical functioning of the human body.

Dr. Still founded the American School of Osteopathic 1892 in Kirksville, Missouri in the United States. After being open for only five years, the school had over 700 students. The doctor even encouraged women and minorities to become professional doctors.

Still and his colleague continually rallied to prove the validity of osteopathic medicine and, finally, in 1973, this persistent paid off. DOs were officially licensed to practice in all American states and were respected of equal capacity and education level as MDs.

## Treating Symptoms vs. Preventing Illness

Prevention is better than cure is the age-old saying, but pharmaceutical companies live by a different code of ethics.

The profits available from prevention are limited, while providing cures has the potential for infinite profits. Modern medicine has taught us to be reactive rather than proactive in our healthcare. We are taught to go to the doctor after we have contracted or developed an illness or disease rather than how to take preventive measures to avoid getting this disease or illness in the first place. When this disease or illness has our health hanging in the balance, then we are prescribed drugs that treat symptoms rather than curing the malady. This is how traditional medicine now works. And this is how so many people get caught in a web of continuous care from MD doctors and the pharmaceutical industry.

This is exactly why it is so important that you choose a DO doctor to provide you with measures that help prevent illness rather than treat symptoms. It is important that you place your healthcare in the hands of someone who does not have a vested interest in ensuring that you remain ill so that they make a profit.

Curing means that after medical treatment a patient no longer suffers from a particular illness or condition anymore. While there has been no progress made in finding a cure for some diseases like Hepatitis B, this is not true all around the board. In cases where the disease is not yet known to be curable, then it does make sense to seek medical treatment to manage the disease so that the symptoms do not affect the patients quality of life to an extent that life seems unbearable. However, in cases such as these, there are many herbal remedies that can aid in fighting the symptoms. Take Hepatitis B, for example. This is a viral disease that causes serious liver infection. The disease is transmitted via infected blood and symptoms can include fever, joint pain, nausea, vomiting, fatigue, and yellowing of the skin and whites of the eyes, which is a condition known as jaundice.

Normally, Hepatitis B is treated with several antiviral medications that are supposed to fight the virus while limiting the damage to the liver. But what of the possible side effects that include hair loss, stomach pain, headaches, diarrhea, sleep problems, vomiting, extreme fatigue and more? These medications are supposed to help such patients but can cause life-threatening effects instead. The use of Epivir, which is one such medication, can lead to a condition known as lactic acidosis. This condition is a buildup of lactic acid in the blood, which leads to blood poisoning and even death.

If these medications have such an extensive list of side effects that can compound the symptoms of this disease and even introduce new ones, why are not doctors telling patients about natural alternatives like milk thistle that offers relief at a much lower expense? Why aren't patients told about the long list of herbs that can help fight liver issues such as Artemisia, mistletoes, kava, nutmeg, valerian root to name just a few?

On the other hand, there are diseases that are curable yet still many patients find themselves having symptoms treated rather than the illness itself. Unfortunately, the common practice is that doctors prescribe medications to manage symptoms rather than the illness. They have been trained to do so–to treat symptoms rather than the underlying issues that perpetuate these illnesses and diseases.

This is where holistic medicine is needed. This type of medicine allows a person to seek optimal health and wellness of the entire person, meaning the body, mind, emotions and spirit. According to the holistic medicine practice, a person can only gain proper balance in life by ensuring all of these areas are performing at optimum levels. The body is made up of interdependent parts, and if one part is not working properly, all the other parts will be affected negatively. Therefore, if a person is in pain and a doctor only prescribed pain medication without looking for the underlying issue that causes the pain, then the imbalance has not been fixed and this person will not be properly healed.

Let us take a look at this example. A patient may walk into a doctor's office complaining of tension headaches. If this person visited a traditional doctor, this doctor will prescribe a medication to treat tension headaches and send the person on their way. More than likely the person will be back with the same symptoms or others because the doctor did not look into the underlying issues that were causing these headaches.

On the other hand, if the person visited a holistic doctor, this doctor would have interviewed the person to look for potential factors that are causing this person's headache. These factors of why can be wide-ranging and could be related to personal problems, stress, poor sleep habits, lack of adequate physical activity, diet and other health problems. The Do's job is to not just hand out prescriptions, but to develop a treatment plan to not only relieve symptoms but to modify the patient's lifestyle to prevent the illness, such as tension headaches, from reoccurring.

Many DO practitioners recommend that patients take responsibility for their own wellness and achieving optimum health. As a result, it is not uncommon for DOs to recommend that a patient educate themselves on making lifestyle changes to promote self-care. These lifestyle changes can include relationship and spiritual counseling, changes in diet and exercise, psychotherapy, and more. The DO may even recommend alternative therapies like homeopathy, massage therapy, acupuncture, and chiropractic care.

# The Doctor's Internal Interest in Prescribing Pharmaceutical Drugs

Many doctors get paid to prescribe pharmaceutical drugs every year. In 2015, doctors in the US alone received payments from pharmaceutical companies and companies in the medical device industry that amounted to 2.4 billion dollars. They received these payments and gifts for encouraging patience to buy pricey brand-name drugs, and this is not where the appalling statistics that show how deeply doctors are into this pharmaceutical companies ends.

Between 2014 and 2015, it was found that several doctors were paid over $25,000 during that time to prescribe opioid. Opioid is a drug with addictive properties that can lead to major psychological effects. It resembles opium and is closely related to the illegal drug called heroin. Opioid is often found in pain relievers such as oxycodone and hydrocodone, both of which are prescription drugs. The doctors who prescribe the most of these opioid prescriptions got paid the most money by these big-name pharmaceutical companies that manufacture the drugs.

This is not the only prescription drug that has been implicated in recent scandals that involve the role of doctors and their interest in the pharmaceutical industry. Doctors are routinely paid to promote pharmaceutical products. This is so severe that the Affordable Care Act was passed in 2010 and requires all pharmaceutical companies to publicly report all payments that were made to doctors that were more than $10. As a result, pharmaceutical companies have had to pay out billions of dollars to settle lawsuits because they were accused of improperly marketing and placing influence on doctors to prescribe medications to patients. More effort has been made to protect patient with the passing of the Physician Payment

Sunshine Act, which is section 6002 of the Affordable Care Act. It requires that pharmaceutical companies disclose any physician ownership or investment interest in these companies.

We go to MD doctors, we believed that they had our best interest at heart. The trust that the public has in MDs continues to crumble with the growing evidence that so many doctors are in the pockets of these big-name pharmaceutical companies. It was found in a nationwide survey in 2009 that more than 80% of doctors have some form of financial interest in pharmaceutical companies. Of this number, 20% received reimbursement for attending medical education events and meetings. That does not leave many doctors on the market that patients can trust. That is truly disheartening!

# How to Choose the Right DO Doctor for You

Your doctor is more than just someone you go to when you feel ill. This person is a confidant who can make a big difference in whether you live your life in good health or in poor condition. You certainly do not want a doctor who continuously prescribes you medication just so that he or she can make a profit by pushing the drugs that pharmaceutical companies design and manufacture down your throat both literally and figuratively.

Here are a few tips you can use to choose the right health care provider for you:

- Ask around for good DO doctors. DO doctors do not have the vested interest in pharmaceutical companies that many MDs do. DO doctors are less likely to prescribe medications, especially pricing medications that just deal with symptoms. These kinds of doctors were taught to treat the whole person, and therefore, focus on how the person can improve their lifestyle to maintain good health.

- Ensure that this doctor is in a convenient location. I am sure that you will not want to travel very far if you are not feeling well to see your doctor. Therefore, ensure that your doctor's office is conveniently located to suit your needs.

- Perform a quality check. Do your research before you go to any doctor. In this day and age, it is simple enough to get on the internet to check on reviews on a doctor. You can even find out if this person keeps up-to-date in the latest developments in the medical field with updated certification.

- Do a cold call. You can tell a lot about a doctor ethic and approach to medicine by phone etiquette of the office staff.

- Keep your needs in mind before you visit any doctor. If you are reading this book then I can assume that you would like a holistic approach to your healthcare. Keep that in mind when you visit the doctor so that you are not swayed in another direction and get placed under the thumb of a doctor's greedy intentions.

- Learn to listen to your gut. We form opinions about other people within seconds of meeting them, but we have been taught to stifle this intuition. Listen to your inner voice, and check to see if your feel at ease with this doctor. Watch how this person behaves. Is he or she kind to his staff and to other patients? Does he or she answer your question and explain things in a way that you clearly understand? Does this person make a concerted effort to listen to your difficulties and concerns? You need to be able to trust your doctor and to talk comfortably with this person. Usually, your gut can tell you whether or not you can trust this person.

# Chapter 4:
# The Holistic Approach

Holistic healing has many stereotypes attached to it. Some people see it as voodoo and magical nonsense that has no sound foundation. However, that is far from the truth. The true definition of holistic healing is the characteristic of comprehending that the human body houses several parts that are intimately interconnected to create a whole body. The whole body functions best when there is synergy between these interrelated parts.

Holistic healing is not just an approach to healthcare. It is an entire lifestyle because your health is not just your body. Your health encompasses your mind and your soul as well. You cannot transform one without transforming the others. Holistic healing is dependent on education so that a person can maintain or restore balance of the mind, body, and soul so that the entire individual can function as a well-maintained and healthy whole.

It is because the ancient Egyptians and the civilizations that came after them recognized the importance of keeping these interconnected parts working in balance that there were such huge strides made in the development of herbal healing. Even Hippocrates was known to promote the power of self-healing. He not only believed that the body had the capability of healing itself from most diseases, but he also encouraged it. Unfortunately, these holistic practices were stifled under the rise of the pharmaceutical industry.

Luckily, this is not an indefinite state of affairs. We as a global society have the power to reclaim control of our bodies and strengthen the body's capabilities to heal itself with what nature has provided us.

Herbal medicine is an essential part of a holistic lifestyle. In this one instance, reliving the past and the way our ancestors approached healthcare can be the way for uplifting the future so that we are healthier and happier.

You can use the engine properties of holistic healing to benefit yourself and become healthier. There are immediate and long-term benefits to exploring this ancient way of healing. Holistic doctors are showing more and more patients how they can challenge the body to open up the mind and spirit so that they can engage their mind for a more fulfilling life. With the guidance of a holistic doctor, you can obtain good life and health for yourself too.

## The Holistic Doctors' Strategy

DOs are just one type of holistic medical practitioner. There are others including integrative physicians, who use a blend of holistic and mainstream medicine; ayurvedic doctors, who use life energy to govern medical practice; and naturopathic doctors, who encourage the body's self-healing abilities to become more prominent. No matter which of these doctors you choose, they all encourage holistic healing practices. All of these doctors promote the attack of the root cause of illness instead of just treating the symptoms. They also aim for preventative medicine and improving overall health.

Holistic medicine also goes by the name of alternative medicine. By Western standards, the advice and healing obtained from alternative medicine is considered untraditional. Despite what is considered the unconventional approach, there is no denying that an increasing number of Americans are finding relief from the illnesses when using the methods prescribed by holistic doctors. Here are a few common alternative medicine techniques that are encouraged by these types of doctors:

- Acupuncture. This is a treatment method with origins in China. This practice is based on the belief that blocked energy centers in the body cause illness and sickness. Thin needles are inserted into specific points on the body by a licensed practitioner to relieve this blockage. Many people who suffer from chronic headaches, chronic back and neck pain, and osteoarthritis have found relief with this technique.

- Chiropractic. This is practice by chiropractors who are licensed doctors trained in spinal adjustment. This has been shown to offer relief from neck pain and headaches.

- Homeopathy. This technique is based on the principle that whatever is causing an illness can be used to treat it. Therefore, practitioners of this method will take a substance that is known to cause harm and dilute it to a near vanishing point to treat an illness. This technique should be approached with extreme caution.

- Meditation. This technique has been used by many people who suffer from mental illnesses, such as anxiety and depression, those who suffer from insomnia and even those who suffer from irritable bowel syndrome. The technique focuses on using deep breathing to center a person to help the mind heal the body from the inside out.

- Massage. Massages are not just great for relaxing but also help with relieving several types of pain, including back pain and pain from injuries.

- Yoga. This is an ancient practice, and it has been around for so long because it has several health benefits, which include reducing blood pressure, easing depression, and relieving lower back pain.

- The use of foods to cure the body. You are what you eat; therefore, holistic doctors encouraged the consumption of healthy and clean foods so that the body becomes clean and healthy. Several foods that are encouraged for consumption include berries for its anti-inflammatory and antioxidant properties; and apple cider vinegar, which helps reduce the risk of cancer, promotes weight loss, help regulate blood sugar and aids in lowering bad cholesterol. Teas and turmeric are common recommendations as well.

- The use of probiotics. Probiotics are the good bacteria in the gut of every human. They not only aid keeping a good balance in the digestive system but also help in maintaining overall health.

- Herbal medicines. Many holistic practices are governed by the fact that the body has several natural self-healing abilities. Holistic doctors work to encourage these abilities to perform better with the air of herbal supplements such as feverfew, which has been shown to decrease the frequency of migraines in some patients, and saw palmetto, which can be used to treat the symptoms of an enlarged prostate.

Other alternative medicine practices include aromatherapy, tai chi, reiki, progressive relaxation, guided imagery, cold water therapy, and hypnotherapy.

## Herbal Remedies and Holistic Healing

Herbal medicine is also called phytomedicine, and its ancient roots have shown us that we can use a plant's flowers, bark, leaves, fruit and roots for medical purposes. The use of herbal medicines can promote the balance of body, mind, and soul and can enhance vitality, promote longevity, and enhance overall health. Herbal medicine has the power to cure, treat, and prevent a wide range of illnesses and diseases from common to rare types. Not only are the benefits far-reaching, but the variety of goods available are astounding. There is a list of several herbs that can aid in maintaining and restoring your overall health. They are listed by the condition that they treat.

## *Anxiety*

This is a mental disorder that is characterized by a general feeling of unease, such as worry or fear. The feelings can range from mild to severe and can affect anyone of any age. There are a few room herbal remedies that can aid in soothing these extreme feelings. They include ashwagandha, lavender, lemon balm, passion fruit, St John's wort, valerian, chamomile and kava kava, which is a plant that is commonly found in the Pacific Islands.

## *Depression*

This is another mental disorder. It is characterized by feelings of dejection and severe sadness. The following herbs can aid in uplift the spirits of those who suffer from this disorder. They include St. John's wort, ginseng, chamomile, lavender, and saffron.

## *High blood pressure*

This is also known as hypertension, and it occurs when the body's blood pressure increases to an unhealthy level. This is calculated by measuring how much blood is passing through blood vessels and the amount of resistance that the blood meets when the heart pumps. Herbal remedies that can aid in reducing hypertension include flaxseed, ginger, garlic, celery seed, basil, cinnamon, cardamom, and cat's claw.

## Migraines

These are characterized by pulsing, throbbing and excruciating pain around the head, neck, and face. The pain can be debilitating. There are herbal remedies that can provide relief. They include ginger, feverfew, coriander seeds, raw potato cuttings, horseradish, yarrow, willow, valerian, rosemary, and lavender.

## Kidney stones

Kidney stones are hard deposits that form in the kidneys. These hard deposits travel through the urinary tract and can cause extreme pain when they exit the body. Herbal remedies that can provide relief include celery seed, wheatgrass, basil, pomegranate, and dandelion.

## High cholesterol

The body does need cholesterol to function optimally; however, there are two types of cholesterol. The good type of cholesterol is known as HDL (high-density lipoprotein) cholesterol, and the bad type of cholesterol is known as LDL (low-density lipoprotein) cholesterol. To keep levels of LDL cholesterol down, the recommended herbal remedies include flaxseed, garlic, hawthorn, green tea, coriander seeds, fenugreek seeds, psyllium husk, and amla.

## Heartburn and acid reflux

Millions of people worldwide suffer from these two conditions, and there are a few herbal remedies that can help in treating the symptoms. They include chamomile, lemon balm, caraway, licorice, peppermint, angelica, and milk thistle.

## Hernia

A hernia is a condition that occurs when an organ pushes through the organ tissue or muscle that holds it in place.

Herbal remedies that can correct this include aloe vera and chamomile.

## Boosting libido

A low sex drive can affect many aspects of a person's life. Luckily, there are herbal remedies, such as the consumption of bananas, figs, and avocados to boost libido. Herbs and other herbal remedies that aid in boosting libido also include ginkgo, ginseng, maca, tribulus terrestris, saffron, fenugreek, and saw palmetto.

## Sore throat

We all know the discomfort and inconvenience of having a sore throat. Luckily, there are herbal remedies that can ease the pain in a shorter period. They include licorice, lemon, ginger, sage, Echinacea, fenugreek, peppermint, and chamomile.

## Common cold and flu

Just like a sore throat, this can be highly inconvenient and uncomfortable to deal with. However, ginger, garlic, and Echinacea are just a few of the herbal remedies that you can use to get the symptoms under control.

## Constipation

If you have a hard time going, try using herbal remedies such as Senna, peppermint, Ginger, dandelion, black or green tea, licorice, or chamomile.

## Menstrual cramps

Turmeric, chaste berry, and black cohosh are just a few of the effective home remedies that can help alleviate the pain of menstruation.

*Menopause*

Herbal remedies such as red clover, dong quai, ginseng, and evening primrose can help give relief of menopausal symptoms.

*Congestion*

Using herbal remedies such as chamomile, green tea, and garlic can clear your nasal passages quickly.

As we go farther into this book, we will touch on some of these herbal remedies in more depth and other ailments that can be cured and prevented with the use of herbal remedies. We will also touch on how a holistic approach to healing can aid in strengthening the immune system, balance hormones, and more.

# Why Insurance Companies Will Not Cover Holistic Treatment

Consumer demand for alternative sources of medicine is at an all-time high, yet there is a resistant to providing patients with insurance coverage when they use natural medicine.

The United States has an expense of 1.5 trillion dollars on healthcare annually, even though most Americans are not satisfied with the healthcare system. This dissatisfaction is why many turn to alternative and natural sources of medicine. Unfortunately, these people have been forced to place their hands in their own pockets to supplement the cost of pursuing a natural medicine to improve their health.

Only a few strides have been made in having insurance companies cover alternative medicine. This includes coverage for chiropractic and acupuncture visits. Almost all other natural treatments are excluded from insurance coverage. This begs the question of why there is a hold up in adding natural medicine coverage to insurance plans, especially when holistic doctors follow the same steps that conventional doctors use.

The answer is obvious. Just as with most other things in the world of medicine, the pharmaceutical industry is causing the stall on this. Pharmaceutical companies do not want to encourage any use of natural medicine, as this will cut into their profits. It is sad to realize, but pharmaceutical companies extend influence even over health insurance. When asked why they do not cover natural medicine, many health companies will say that there is not enough evidence to prove the effectiveness of natural medicine even after centuries of proof has been provided. Insurance companies claim that they do not want to take on the risk of supporting a medicine that has not been proven as a form of treatment. Simply put, they do not want to pay for a treatment that they are not sure is valid. The plain truth is that unhealthy and ill people pay more in insurance because they expect the worst.

Insurance companies have a vested interest in keeping you sick as well. A lot less people would not carry insurance if they did not foresee major illness in their future.

It is clear to see that we as a global society cannot depend on the pharmaceutical industry or even health insurance companies to watch out for our best interests. We have to take on that responsibility ourselves. Educating yourself is the first step to taking that power back from these big-name companies. This book can help you to nourish your mind with the facts so that you can achieve that whole body balance.

# Chapter 5:
# Your Immune System

## What is the Immune System?

The immune system is a complex network made up of organs, tissues, and cells that fight infections from bacteria, viruses, parasites and fungi, and set up systems to deal with infections should they manage to occur. The immune system is the body's natural defense system against cells that are bad for it.

These invaders can come from several sources, such as breathing in these invasive cells, ingesting contaminated food or water, or through physical contact, such as touching skin or having sex, and even through the eyes. These invasive cells can also get into the body through shared needles and insect bites.

The immune system uses several lines of defense to block out these invaders. Such defensive measures include:

- The skin, which is a waterproof barrier that secretes oil and contains cell properties that suppress and kill invasive cells.
- The digestive tract, which is lined with a mucous layer that contains more of these cells and properties. The digestive tract also contains acid in the stomach, which can kill invasive cells as well.
- The lungs, which are lined with a mucous layer to trap foreign entities. This mucus layer is moved upward by small hair-like structures so that it can be coughed out to remove any trapped invasive species.

- Saliva and tears contain antibacterial enzymes that help reduce the risk of foreign entities entering the body.

These are only a few of the defenses that the body has in place to keep harmful invasive species away.

The body is good at preventing repeated infections when these invasive species do manage to get through by remembering the properties of these invasive species so that it can be ready to defend the body faster the next time. This is facilitated by special cells known as memory cells that recognize and destroy microbes quickly when they enter the body again. The invasive infections knowns as the flu and common cold change the makeup of their cells often, which is why human beings have a hard time preventing the contraction of these infections.

## The Parts of the Immune System

The immune system is made up of several parts. They include:

- White blood cells. These are manufactured in the bone marrow and are part of the lymphatic system. They travel throughout the body through the blood and tissues looking for invasive cells so that they can launch an immune attack when the find these invaders. There are several types of white blood cells.

- Antibodies. Antibodies are crucial to the immune defense of the body. They recognize substances that are called antigens on the surface of microbes, or the chemicals that the microbes produce that mark them as foreign to the body. When the cells recognize these antigens, they mark the cells for destruction and as such as cells, proteins, and other chemicals move in for this attack.

- The complement system. This system is made up of special proteins that work in conjunction with antibodies to mark and destroy foreign entities.

- The lymphatic system. This is a complex system made up of delicate tubes that run throughout the body. The system is made up of lymph nodes that trap foreign entities; lymph vessels that are tubes that carry lymph, a colorless liquid that bathes the body tissues and contains white blood cells; and white blood cells, which are also called lymphocytes. The lymphatic system aids the immune system by managing the fluid levels throughout the body, reacting to the presence of foreign entities, locating and destroying cancerous cells, locating and destroying cell products that can lead to diseases or disorders, and absorbing some of the fat from our diets from the intestines.

- The bone marrow. This is a spongy tissue that is found inside of our bodies. It manufactures several cells, including the red blood cells that are needed to carry oxygen throughout the body; the white blood cells that are used to fight infection; and platelets, which we need for our blood to clot in the event that we sustain an injury.

- The spleen. This organ is responsible for blood filtering and aids in the removal of foreign cells in addition to destroying old or damaged red blood cells. It is also responsible for making components like antibodies and lymphocytes.

- Thymus. This aids in producing white blood cells called T-lymphocytes and also monitors and filters blood content.

## Disorders of the Immune System

Sometimes the function of the immune system can be exaggerated beyond what is needed. One such exaggeration includes allergic reactions and diseases. Allergic reactions are defenses the immune system uses in response to allergens that are overly strong. These include allergies to medication, food, and insect bites. Another such example is known as anaphylaxis, a severe allergic reaction that can lead to death in response to throat or tongue swelling, shortness of breath, lightheadedness, vomiting and low blood pressure. Examples of overreactions of the immune system include asthma, hives, dermatitis, eczema, sinus disease, and hay fever.

Another example of over-activity of the immune system is autoimmune diseases. Such diseases include type 1 diabetes, rheumatoid arthritis, and multiple sclerosis. Autoimmune diseases arise when the immune system mounts a defense against normal functions of the body.

The immune system can also underreact in a condition called immunodeficiency. This under-activity makes people vulnerable to infections that can be life-threatening. Immunodeficiency can arise due to genetics, medical treatment such as the use of pharmaceutical drugs, such as corticosteroids and chemotherapy, or be caused by other diseases, such as HIV/AIDS.

## How Processed Foods and Pharmaceutical Drugs Can Negatively Affect the Immune System

As the saying goes, "You are what you eat" and this applies to your immune system. Consuming a lot of processed food can sabotage your immune system. The first reason this can occur is because consuming too many processed foods can lead to poor gut health. There is a delicate balance of good and bad bacteria living in your digestive system. The good bacteria break down food, aid in the absorption of nutrients, and help keep toxic materials out of your body. These good bacteria rely on a good supply of vitamins and minerals to keep them in good working order. Consuming the huge supply of sugar, salt, and unhealthy fats that are obtained in processed food throws off the fine balance of this entire ecosystem.

This allows the growth of bad bacteria and yeast, which overpowers the presence of good bacteria. This compromises the function of the immune system not only because these microbes are already present in the body but also because the function of keeping other microbes out of the body is compromised. The only way to avoid these issues is to drastically reduce the consumption of processed foods so that you can eliminate toxins from your diet. They should be replaced with healthy options that provide the body with healthy nutrition and the probiotics it needs to maintain the healthy balance of microbes in the gut.

Secondly, consuming processed food increases inflammation in the body. This arises as a response from the immune system to deal with the consumption of too much sugar, salt, and unhealthy fats. The more the body is bombarded with processed food, the more the immune system overreacts and increases inflammation. Chronic inflammation can impair the function of the immune system severely.

This can be reversed by consuming less processed foods and consuming more anti-inflammatory foods, such as tomatoes, olive oil, fruits, nuts, green leafy vegetables and fish, such as salmon and tuna.

The immune system is not only weakened by the consumption of processed foods but possibly by the pharmaceutical drugs that you take. Some pharmaceutical medications contain a dangerous side effect, which is weakening of the immune system. This places you at risk of developing several infections, all in the name of fighting off one illness. These are called immunosuppressant drugs. There are several types of immunosuppressant drugs and they include:

- Corticosteroids. These are typically used to provide relief from inflammation in certain parts of the body. Popular types include prednisone, Deltasone and Orasone, budesonide, and prednisolone.
- Janus kinase inhibitors. These are a type of drug that works by inhibiting the activities of certain hormones that are needed to facilitate the function of the immune system. An example is tofacitinib.
- IMDH inhibitors. These suppress the synthesis of adhesive reception that are needed to regulate cell-to-cell contact. This can inhibit the role of white blood cells and antibodies. Examples include azathioprine, leflunomide, and mycophenolate.

Other drugs that inhibit the functions of the immune system are biologics, mTOR inhibitors, TNF inhibitors, and calcineurin inhibitors.

It is ironic that doctors prescribe these medications in a bid to help you become healthier, but these same medications put you are risk for infections that can impair your health more.

# How to Maintain a Healthy Immune System

Now that we have established how important the immune system is to good health, here are a few ways you can ensure that yours remains strong:

- Ensure that you are getting enough sleep. Getting the right amount and good quality sleep is as essential to maintaining a healthy body as eating and breathing are. Adults typically requires seven to nine hours of sleep nightly to reap several health benefits, one of which is a strengthened immune system.

- Eat less sugar. Consuming sugars slows down the function of the immune system; therefore, its attack to fighting foreign entities. Substitute sugar for healthier alternatives such as plant-based stevia and maple syrup.

- Practice deep breathing techniques. We breathe unconsciously, but the impact that breathing has on our overall health is great. Getting enough oxygen fuels you with energy and a lack of proper supply contributes to many health issues such as the development of cancer, heart disease, digestive problems, aching joints, and respiratory problems.

- Eat more fermented food. Examples of fermented foods include miso, kimchi, tempeh, sauerkraut, and yogurt. Fermented foods contain enzymes and probiotics that are not only aid in improving the function of the digestive system but also strengthening the immune system.

- Spend more time outdoors. Spending time basking in the sun provides your body with the much-needed Vitamin D, which plays a vital role in supporting the immune system.

- Do a detox diet. Unfortunately, we live in a world that is filled with pollution and many individuals consume substances that introduce toxins into their bodies on a daily basis. These substances include caffeine, sugar, alcohol, gluten, dairy, and the chemicals found in processed foods. A detox diet aids in removing these toxins from the body by promoting the consumption of whole grains, vegetables, and fruits. In addition to removing toxins from the body, these foods provide needed nutrition that aids in strengthening the immune system.

- Practice stress relieving techniques. Stress suppresses the function of a healthy immune system. Laugh more, practice yoga, meditate and find other ways of enjoying life so that your immune system can work better.

- Increase your antioxidant intake. Antioxidants help strengthen the immune system so consuming more antioxidant-rich foods and drinks such as dark chocolate, blueberries, and green tea should be a priority.

## Plant-Based Foods That Help to Boost the Function of the Immune System

The way that you eat determines whether your immune system is strong or weakened. Here are a few fruits and vegetables that you can consume to strengthen your immune system:

- Citrus fruits. There is a long list of citrus fruits, and this list includes oranges, tangerines, lemons, limes and grapefruits. These foods are rich in vitamin C, and vitamin C increases the production of white blood cells, which is key for fighting off infections and boosting the function of the immune system. Unfortunately, the body does not store or produce vitamin C so continuous consumption is required to ensure that levels remain at optimum.

- Red bell peppers. These contain twice as much vitamin C as citrus fruits. They also contain beta carotene, which helps to keep your skin and eyes healthy.

- Garlic. Garlic contains heavy concentration of sulfur-rich compounds that aid in strengthening the immune system. Garlic also helps lower blood pressure and slow down the hardening of blood arteries.

- Ginger. Ginger is a food that you can use in the aftermath of an infection, such as the common cold or the flu to help decrease inflammation, soothe a sore throat, and decrease nausea.

- Broccoli. This food is packed with vitamins, minerals, fiber, and antioxidants. Ensure that it is cooked as little as possible to reap the most benefit.

- Spinach. This is packed with beta carotene, vitamin C, and antioxidants. Again, this is a vegetable that should be cooked as little as possible to get the most nutritional value from it.

- Green and black tea. Both of these teas are rich in flavonoids, which are a type of antioxidant. Green tea is also a good source of an amino acid called L-theanine. This amino acid is needed for the production of lymphocytes.

- Papaya. This fruit is loaded with vitamin C and also has a digestive enzyme called papain, which has anti-inflammatory properties.

- Kiwi. This contains high levels of vitamin C.

- Sunflower seeds. These contain several vitamins and minerals, one of which is vitamin E, which is a powerful antioxidant.

- Avocado. This contains high levels of vitamin E.

- Dark green leafy. They also contain high levels of vitamin E.
- Almonds. This is another food that contains high levels of vitamin E.

# Chapter 6:
# Cleanse and Rejuvenate Your Body

We live in a world that is filled with pollution. It is in our food, in the air that we breathe, the things that we touch, and more. Our bodies were designed to naturally detoxify and remove these toxins but with such a high level of pollution, our bodies can become overburdened easily and needs help in the detoxification process.

Detoxification has been used for centuries by different cultures around the world to maintain and renew optimum health, to feed the body, to maintain health and nutrition and to protect the body from disease. These past centuries of knowledge can help you achieve the same for your body.

## What is a Detox?

This is a short-term diet intervention designed to eliminate toxins from the body. There are several ways to detoxify the body, and we will discuss a few common methods below. But first let's take a moment to speak on what a detox does for the body. A detox:

- Helps improve blood circulation
- Provides the body with healthy nutrition
- Stimulates the liver to get rid of toxins
- Helps restore the body organs
- Promotes the elimination of toxins through sweat urine and feces

# Reasons Why You Need to Detox

Not sure if you need a detox? Here are a few signs that your body may be giving you that it is crying out for one:

- You often feel lacking in energy, fatigued, and a general feeling of being unwell. A detox diet is said to help you feel more alive, happy, and full of energy because it is the presence of these toxins that often has a person feeling brain fog, body achiness, digestive issues, headaches, allergies, and other issues that generally bring us down.

- You often suffer from sugar and carb cravings. Carbohydrates are used by the body to generate energy. Sugars are the simplest form of carbohydrates. Initially when carbohydrates are consumed, we experience a rush of energy that makes us feel invincible at times but soon after we experienced an energy crash. Unfortunately, when we consume sugar, it stimulates the reward center of our brains, which makes us crave more sugar to get over the sugar crash. The stimulation of the reward center of the brain by sugar makes it an addictive substance. Excessive sugar intake leads to several negative health benefits, including obesity, the development of cardiovascular diseases, type 2 diabetes, kidney and liver problems, and more

- You suffer from issues of weight loss. If you cannot lose weight and keep it off, this may be a sign that your body is in need of a diet to get rid of toxins in addition to eating healthier. Most of the weight loss management issues we have arise because we practice a diet that is rich in processed foods that carry empty calories and do not have the nutrition that our bodies need. This can lead to weight gain. In addition, these processed foods are often high in sugar, which is an addictive substance. Excessive sugar intake triggers insulin spikes and inflammation, both of which are conditions that make it hard to maintain a healthy weight.

Other reasons include:

- You have never detoxed. Detoxifying should be done at least once a year.
- You often suffer from allergies
- You often suffer from low-grade infection
- You are often bloated
- You suffer from menstrual problems
- You often suffer from irritated skin
- You often feel mentally confused
- You have puffy eyes or bags underneath the eyes

## How Does Detoxing Work?

Detoxifying sounds like a complicated process, when in actuality it is quite simple. The process of detoxification removes impurities in the blood by delivering them to the liver where they are processed for elimination. These toxins can also be eliminated through the lungs, intestines, kidneys, lymphatic system, and skin. The body has systems in place to deal with impurities and toxins, but when they are not properly filtered, the body is adversely affected. This is why detoxifying is such a valuable process to partake in.

## Benefits of Detoxing

Detoxification is an important component of maintaining optimum health, and here are just a few benefits that you will be rewarded with when you detoxify your body:

- Reduced inflammation
- Healthier and improved appearance of skin
- Healthier Fuller hair
- Strengthened immune system
- Boosted energy levels
- Better weight management
- Improved performance of digestive system
- Better smelling breath
- Improved mood and mental health
- Improved focus and concentration
- Increased longevity

# Common Ways of Detoxing

### The Smoothie Cleanse Detox Diet

This detox diet is based on replacing the regular meals of breakfast, lunch, and dinner with nutritionally balanced smoothies made from whole plant-based ingredients. This detox diet follows the following rules:

- There is to be no consumption of seafood, cheese, meat, processed foods, alcohol, or bread.
- Three smoothies shall be consumed daily with two snacks in between.
- At least 12 glasses of water should be drank daily.
- 30+ minutes of physical exercise is required daily.
- This diet should be practiced for at least five days.

### Easy Detoxifying Smoothie Recipes

To help get you started on your smoothie cleanse, here are a few ingredients mixes that you can use. All you need is a blender. Throw in the ingredients and blend until a smooth, uniform consistency is attained. To ensure that your smoothie has balanced nutrition, here are a few guidelines to follow:

- Add at least one handful of green leafy vegetables such as spinach, kale, or bok choy.
- Ensure that you get your fiber by adding oats, chia seeds, or flax seeds.
- Add healthy fats like avocado, nut butters, or coconut oil or butter
- Obtain your protein requirement by adding protein powder, Greek yogurt or nut butters.
- Liquid bases such as coconut milk, almond milk, and unsweetened fruit juice can be added.
- Use water or ice to smoothen out the smoothie without adding calories.
- Honey or maple syrup can be used as a natural sweetener, but ingredients such as yogurt, fruit, and nut butter are already sweetened so you may not need to add a sweetener.

Without further ado, here are the ingredient list for tasty smoothies that can be prepared in five minutes or less and are one serving.

**Almond Zucchini Smoothie**

- 1 yellow zucchini, chopped
- 2 tablespoons of almond butter
- 1 pear
- 1 cup of almond milk
- 1 cup of spinach

- 1/2 teaspoon of cinnamon
- 1/2 cup of water

**Berry Spinach Smoothie**

- 1 cup of mixed berries
- 3 tablespoons of almond butter
- 1 cup of almond milk
- 3 tablespoons of Greek yogurt
- 2 stalks kale with the ends chopped off
- 1/2 teaspoon of honey
- 3 tablespoons of chia seeds

**Green Grapefruit Smoothie**

- 1 cup spinach
- 1/2 avocado
- 1/2 tablespoon of grated Ginger
- 1 cup of chilled green tea
- 1 small banana
- 1 scoop vanilla protein powder
- 1/2 tablespoon of lime juice

**Ginger Carrot Smoothie**

- 1 large carrot, chopped
- 1 tablespoon of grated Ginger
- 1/2 teaspoon of turmeric powder
- 1 chopped pear
- 2 kale stalks with the ends dropped off
- 1 tablespoon of coconut oil

- 1 tablespoon of flax seeds
- 1 cup of ice

**Matcha Almond Smoothie**

- 1 teaspoon of matcha powder
- 4 tablespoon of almond butter
- 1 cup spinach
- 1 avocado
- 1 pear
- 1/2 teaspoon of vanilla extract
- 1 cup of almond milk

**Snacking on the Smoothie Cleanse Detox Diet**

When snacking on this detox diet, snacks should be limited to 200 calories or less. To keep things interesting, you can have a different snack every time. Some great snack options include:

- Seeds and nuts
- Veggie chips
- Dehydrogenated fruit
- Chopped veggies with guacamole or nut butters such as almond butter, peanut butter and cashew butter
- Greek yogurt
- Granola

*The Simple Fruit and Veggie Detox*

This detox diet promotes the consumption of fruits and vegetables only for three days. This detox plan is particularly attractive to people who would like to lose weight fast and conquer food addiction quickly. The basic rules are:

- Drink at least 12 glasses of water every day
- Do not drink any non-water beverages including tea and coffee
- Eat only fresh fruits that are preferably organic. No canned, frozen, or dried fruits allowed.
- Have a salad with non-starchy organic vegetables in the evening
- Avoid exercising
- Supplemental protein drinks can be consumed

## *Juice Cleanse Detox Diet*

This detox diet involves consuming only juices from fruits and vegetables as a means of detoxifying the body and losing weight. Juicing involves squeezing the juice from vegetables and fruits while separating them from the pulp. This is different from blending, which includes mixing all the edible parts of the vegetables and fruits, including the pulp. This detox method is controversial as it restricts several food groups and calories. However, many people swear by its benefits.

The rules for following this detox diet include:

- It must be done for a period ranging from 3 to 10 days
- The practitioner must drink only liquids and juices for the detox.
- Dietary supplements must be taken in combination to juicing.
- Juicing can be combined with other colon cleansing methods such as colonic irrigation or enemas

## The Benefits of Practicing the Juice Clean Detox Diet

- Obtaining high amounts of vitamins and minerals

- Boosted immune system
- Boosted energy
- Decreased risk of inflammation
- Improved digestion
- Lowered blood sugar levels
- Improved nutrient absorption
- Aids in lowering bad cholesterol levels
- Faster weight loss
- Helps boosts athletic performance

To help you gain these benefits, here is a list of fruits and vegetables that can be juiced in combinations to provide maximum efficiency in the detoxing process:

- Spinach. This has anti-cancer properties and is packed in vitamins. Its mild flavor can be disguised by adding other ingredients.
- Kale. Kale is a powerful antioxidant and anti-inflammatory agent. It also aids in relieving the symptoms of arthritis and autoimmune diseases.
- Cucumber. This vegetable is made of 95% water and has powerful functions in detoxifying the kidney and liver.
- Carrots. This aids in improving eye health and lowering cholesterol in addition to being a good source of fiber, potassium, Vitamin K, and beta carotene.
- Beets. This also helps fight inflammation and lowers blood pressure.
- Celery. This has a high water content and is a good source of fiber, Vitamin K, Vitamin C, and Vitamin A.
- Ginger. This aids in supporting a healthy immune

system and digestive system.

- Oranges. In addition to being high in Vitamin C and low in calories, this is an immune system booster.
- Apples. This aids in supporting cardiovascular health and is an anti-inflammatory agent.
- Lemon. This is a highly effective cleansing agent and cuts through the bitterness of using greens like kale.

## Juicing Recipes

Below you will find a list of ingredients for tasty and highly detoxifying recipes. Remember that all vegetables and fruits need to be washed thoroughly before use and cut into ½-inch chunks. All peels should be removed. A high-quality juicer should be used, and the veggies and fruits should be juiced according to the manufacturer's instructions. All of these recipes can be served at room temperature or chilled.

### Carrot Spinach Juice Recipe

- 4 small carrots
- 1 cup of spinach
- 1 cup of parsley
- ½ apple

This recipe is great for achieving clear skin.

### Green Juice Recipe

- 1 lemon
- 1 inch size piece fresh ginger
- 2 green apples
- 4 kale leaves
- 1 small cucumber

- 1 celery stalk

**Pink Grapefruit Juice Recipe**

- 1 pink grapefruit
- 2 oranges
- 1 head romaine lettuce
- 4 mint leaves

This detoxifying juice recipe promotes weight loss.

**The Ultimate Green Apple Detox Juice Recipe**

- 2 green apples
- 2 celery stalks with no leaves
- 1 small cucumber
- 6 kale leaves
- 1 inch piece fresh ginger
- ½ lemon

**Red Breakfast Juice Recipe**

- 2 beets
- 2 apples
- 2 carrots
- 2 lemons

## *Sugar Detox Diet*

This detox diet involves limiting the amount of sugar that is consumed daily. Practicing this diet is intended to purge the body of unhealthy sugar. This diet can be practiced for a few days, but the practitioner cannot simply revert to consuming sugars indiscriminately after a few days have passed. As a result, some people choose to permanently practice this diet.

## Types of Sugar

Sugar comes in different forms and they include:

**Fructose**

This is the type of sugar that is naturally found in fruit. Even though consuming fruits is healthy, consuming too much fructose can have a negative impact on your health. This negative impact arises because fructose is broken down in the liver, which turns this into compounds such as triglycerides that can cause damage to the liver, free radicals that can damage body cells, and uric acid that can damage the arteries.

**Sucrose**

This is the type of sugar commonly referred to as table sugar. It is the type of sugar that is added to baked goods, candy, and most other sugary foods that we consume. This sugar is a combination of fructose and another type of sugar called glucose. When the sugar is broken down into these two individual parts, glucose causes a spike in blood sugar levels.

**Glucose**

This is the sugar molecule that the body commonly uses to derive energy. Glucose does not need to be consumed because the body naturally breaks down carbohydrates to form the molecule. Having too much glucose in the system causes an unhealthy rise in blood sugar levels.

**High fructose corn syrup**

This is made from cornstarch and is composed of glucose and fructose just like sucrose.

## Why is a Sugar Detox Necessary?

This is not an easy diet to undergo, simply because sugar is an addictive substance. However, it is worth limiting its consumption because it has been linked to a number of medical conditions such as type 2 diabetes, heart disease, mental illness, and obesity.

Because sugar is such a highly addictive substance, people will experience withdrawal symptoms when practicing the sugar detox diet. Mental withdrawal symptoms include depression, anxiety, problems focusing and concentrating, changes in sleep pattern, and sugar cravings. Physical withdrawal symptoms include lightheadedness, dizziness, fatigue, nausea, and tingling of the skin.

To fight this withdrawal symptoms, here are a few tips you can employ:

- Quit sugar cold turkey
- Increase your fiber intake
- Eat more protein
- Avoid using artificial sweeteners
- Get rid of junk food and processed foods in your home
- Drink more water
- Exercise regularly
- Manage your stress levels
- Consumer green vegetables
- Get good quality and quantity sleep

**Health benefits of Decreased Sugar Consumption**

- Improved dental health
- Decreased risk of developing cardiovascular diseases
- Improved focus and concentration
- Lowered blood sugar; therefore, lower the risk of developing type 2 diabetes

- Weight loss
- Reduced inflammation
- Boosted energy
- More mindful eating

**How to Practice the Sugar Detox Diet**

Remember that the first few days of the sugar detox diet can be trying due to sugar withdrawal and its associated symptoms, but with some effort you can make it through to the healthier side. Here are a few tips you can employ to make your sugar detox diet a success:

- Consume at least 45 grams of protein when you eat breakfast. This will allow you to feel full throughout the day.
- Include protein in every meal that you eat. Healthy protein options include eggs, fish, and plant-based sources like beans and tofu.
- Limit the amount of red meat that you consume.
- Do not consume processed meats like bacon and cold cuts.
- Include green leafy vegetables in every meal.
- Include between 45 and 75 grams of healthy fats such as avocado, salmon, flaxseeds, olive, and olive oil every day.
- Limit the consumption of fruits.
- Avoid processed foods such as crackers and chips

# Additional Ways to Help Your Body Detox

After you have practice whatever detoxification method that

you chose, be sure to keep your body cleansed by following the practices mentioned below:

- Eat more foods with Vitamin C or take a supplement. This vitamin helps the body produce a compound in the liver that drives toxins away. This compound is called glutathione.
- Drink the recommended number of glasses of water every day. This allows the better transport of nutrients to the different parts of your body in addition to eliminating false hunger and hydrating your cells.
- Practice deep breathing technique to ensure that oxygen circulates completely throughout your body.
- Manage your stress levels by managing your work/home life, practicing meditation techniques like yoga, and being grateful every day.
- Eat a lot of fiber through plant-based sources, such as beets, radishes, broccoli and artichokes.
- Keep the liver cleansed by drinking green tea and consuming herbs like dandelion root and milk thistle.
- Sweat in the sauna so that your body can eliminate toxins through perspiration.
- Get plenty of exercise so that your body can detoxify itself through perspiration.
- Remove toxins through your pores by dry brushing your skin or trying detoxifying foot spas and baths.
- Practice hydrotherapy. This is the practice of taking a very warm shower for five minutes and allowing the water to run down your back. This is followed up by allowing cold water to wash over your body for 30 seconds. Repeat this three times then get into bed for 30

minutes.

- Limit alcohol intake.
- Limit caffeine intake. Drinking caffeinated drink brings your body to a more acidic state. Decreasing the intake allows the body to be more alkaline, which is more conducive to detoxing.

Be sure to consult your doctor before you start practicing any detox diet.

# Chapter 7:
# Plant-Based Diet

With the word "diet" being thrown around so easily these days, it can seem overwhelming when choosing the one that is right for you. With the many benefits that plants afford us medicinally, it only makes sense to try a plant-based diet to reap the benefits of such clean eating. However, before we delve into the topic of plant-based eating, let's take a look at processed foods and why they are bad for your health.

## What are Processed Foods?

A processed food is any food that has been altered in some way during the preparation process to make it more flavorful, convenient, or shelf-stable. There are various degrees of processing foods.

*Types of Food Processing*

The NOVA classification system, which was introduced in 2009, lists food processing in four categories. They are:

- Unprocessed or minimally processed foods. These foods are still in their natural state by the end of the processing. Unprocessed foods are naturally edible parts of a plant or animal. Minimally processed foods are altered slightly. This is usually done to extend the shelf-life of the foods. For example, pre-cut green beans are processed foods; however, they look almost the same as you would find them in nature. Processes that alter minimally processed foods include cleaning, freezing, vacuum-packaging, refrigerating, pasteurization, and fermentation.

- Processed culinary ingredients. These are food ingredients that are derived from minimally-processed foods through processes such as refining, pressing, and grinding. These ingredients are not usually eaten on their own by used to prepare other dishes. They include plant-based oils, flour, pasta made from whole grains, seeds, and nuts.

- Processed foods. There are foods that are from either of the first two categories to which fat, sugar, or salt has been added. There are usually ready to eat without preparation and contain at least two ingredients. Examples included canned fish, canned fruits, and some cheeses.

- Heavily processed foods. These are also called ultra-processed foods. They have been chemically altered with additives, artificial flavors, and other ingredients. They are prepared beyond the addition of fat, sugar, and salt. Examples include chips, cookies, and some frozen dinner and breakfast cereals. Highly-processed foods pose the highest danger to health because they were prepared with ingredients made to increase cravings and overeating.

**Properties of Highly-Processed Foods**

- They are usually filled with sugar, which can go by other names such as high fructose corn syrup. While our bodies do use sugars to gain energy, most of these added sugars are empty calories that contain no real nutritional value. In addition, consuming too much sugar can lead to devastating health consequences, such as unhealthy weight gain and increased risk of developing cardiovascular diseases. Also, sugar is a highly addictive substance. In fact, sugar is almost ten times as addictive as cocaine. This is why we find it so hard to keep away from sugars and junk food in general.

- They are usually stripped of fiber. Fiber helps us feel full faster, which allows us to consume fewer calories. Fiber also helps with the absorption of carbohydrates. The lack of fiber in highly processed foods makes these foods go through the digestive system quicker, which makes it more difficult for the body to feel satisfied. This leads to the consumption of larger meals and more frequent meals, which leads to unhealthy weight gain in addition to other negative health consequences.

- They usually contain additives. An additive is a substance that is added to food to alter its taste, appearance, or shelf life. Unfortunately, these additives stimulate the reward system in the brain by activating the release of the neurotransmitter called dopamine. Dopamine is a feel-good hormone that makes the person attached to these processed foods. This attachment makes it harder to stop eating them.

- They typically contain several ingredients that are hard to pronounce. These ingredients are artificial and are used to enhance flavor, extended shelf-life or improve the texture of the product. The terms are even masked by generating names such as artificial flavor.

- They can contain high levels of sodium. Salt is added to highly-processed food to improve the taste and texture and increase shelf-life. While the body does need sodium to function at optimum capacity, too much salt can increase sodium levels in the blood to an unsafe level and elevate the risk of developing cardiovascular diseases and high blood pressure.

- Highly processed foods are typically extremely low in nutritional value compared to unprocessed or minimally processed foods. This is because the processing procedure strips these foods of their nutritional value. Even though synthetic minerals and vitamins are added to replace those lost during the process of manufacturing these goods, they cannot compare to the original nutrients.

- They often contain trans fats and processed oils. This is because they are often manufactured with refined seed and vegetable oils that are hydrogenated. This is done because it is a cheap alternative that increases the shelf-life of these foods. Trans fats are unhealthy to consume and can lead to inflammation and unhealthy weight gain.

**The Health Risk Associated With Eating Heavily Processed Foods**

- Highly processed foods can alter moods. Most people have heard of the term hangry, which is an emotionally aggressive state that some people suffer from when they are hungry or deprived of a particular snack or food. This is because of the addictive nature of processed food, which increases irritability and aggression. In addition, consuming highly processed foods contributes to the development of mental illnesses such as anxiety and depression.

- Processed foods can disrupt the consumer's sleep patterns. Consuming too many sugars and salts make it hard to fall asleep and stay asleep. This is because of the energy spikes and crashes that are related to fluctuating blood sugar and insulin levels.

- Processed foods increase the risk of becoming obese. Because processed foods are easy to grab, addictive in nature and do not make us feel as full. this usually leads to overeating. This can lead to unhealthy weight gain, which can lead to obesity. Obesity is a disease that develops from having too much body fat. Obesity is different from being overweight, which can mean that a person simply weighs too much. Bones, fat, and retained water can contribute to a person being overweight. Obesity is not a disease that happens in isolation but occurs in conjunction with a host of other diseases such as diabetes, heart disease, and certain cancers.
- Consuming highly-processed food increases the risk of developing certain types of cancer.
- Eating highly-processed foods increases the risk of developing metabolic diseases, such as diabetes and irritable bowel syndrome.

### *How to Reduce the Amount of Processed Foods in Your Diet*

Because processed foods are available in such a high number and variety, it is difficult for the everyday man and woman to avoid them. However, there are a few practices that you can use to reduce the amount of processed foods that you consume on a daily basis. These practices include:

- Checking the labels of the foods that you purchase. Typically processed foods have a longer ingredients list compared to minimally or unprocessed foods. They also typically have ingredients that are hard to pronounce. Watch out for these, and try to stick to foods that have a short list of ingredients and ingredients that you can pronounce and are familiar with.

- Keep food shopping at grocery stores to a minimum. Whole food markets at a great area to locate minimally or unprocessed foods. Typically grocery stores stock tons of packaged foods that are highly processed.

- Try to avoid highly processed meats such as bacon and sausage, and choose minimally-processed meats such as seafood and chicken breast.

- Cook at home more often. This gives you more control of your diet compared to eating out at restaurants. To make this easier to do, you can cook in batches and keep your meals frozen so that you can dine on tasty leftovers any day of the week.

- Practice a food plant-based diet. Plant-based diets revolve around eating foods that are derived from plants while keeping processed foods to a minimum if they are not avoided altogether.

## What is a Plant-Based Diet?

A plant-based diet is one that emphasizes the consumption of whole vegetables and fruits and whole grains while minimizing the intake of processed foods and animal products. It is a common misconception that a plant-based diet is one that is either vegan or vegetarian. While there are many similarities between the three diets, they are not synonymous.

Those who follow the vegan diet abstain from consuming animal products, including eggs, honey, seafood and dairy. On the other hand, vegetarians exclude all meat and poultry from their diets but still consume some animal products, such as dairy, eggs and seafood. A plant-based diet, on the other hand, offers more flexibility. While practitioners consume mostly plant products, animal products are not completely off-limit, even though the practitioner may choose to exclude all animal products or consume only small amounts of meat, dairy, eggs, poultry, and seafood. The beauty of this diet is that it holds no strict guidelines. The only rule is that the practitioner focuses on eating fresh foods derived from plant sources and minimizing processed and animal-based foods.

## What Can be Eaten on the Plant-Based Diet

Since the plant-based diet is so flexible, many people find that they can eat a lot of foods that they enjoyed before. Even if it is dramatically different, such as in cases where the person consumed mostly processed foods, then I have made locating the things that you can and cannot eat a cinch. This list can double as a shopping list.

## Plant-Based Shopping List

### Fruits

These include pears, mangoes, bananas, pineapple, oranges, limes, lemons, tangerines, berries, peaches, grapes, plums, watermelon, jackfruit, cantaloupe, avocados, apples, cherries, honeydew, and kiwi.

### Dried fruits

Dried fruits include raspberries, raisins, prunes, dates, apricots, and mango.

### Vegetables

Vegetables include cauliflower, broccoli, squash, eggplant, zucchini, tomatoes, spinach, kale, carrots, asparagus, peppers, sweet potatoes, potatoes, eggplant, celery, radish, onions, mushrooms, cucumber, cabbage, Brussel sprouts, artichoke hearts, turnips, lettuce, collard greens, arugula, bok choy, beets, yams, pumpkins, corn, and parsnip.

### Whole grains

These include rolled oats, quinoa, brown rice, whole grain pasta, barley, farro, couscous, cornmeal, rye, buckwheat, millet, spelt, bulgur, and whole grain tortillas.

### Seeds and nuts

These include almonds, cashews, macadamia, pumpkin seeds, sunflower seeds, Brazil nuts, Hazelnuts, Flaxseeds, pine nuts, sesame seeds, pecans, hemp seeds, chia seeds, walnuts, and teff.

### Nut butters

Nut butters include tahini, cashew butter, peanut butter, macadamia butter, pistachio butter, hazelnut butter, almond butter, walnut butter, and pecan butter.

### Plant-based milks

These include coconut milk, almond milk, cashew milk, and soymilk.

### Plant-based proteins

These include tofu, edamame, and tempeh.

### Healthy fats

Healthy fats include olive oil, coconut oil, avocado oil, unsweetened coconut, grapeseed oil, rice bran oil, coconut butter, canola oil, and macadamia oil.

### Legumes and beans

These include chickpeas, lentils, peanuts, black beans, black-eye peas, kidney beans, lima beans, whites beans, pinto beans, mung beans, and garbanzos.

## Sweeteners

Sweeteners include beet sugar, dates, coconut sugar, agave nectar, brown rice syrup, maple syrup, stevia, raw cane sugar, palm sugar, and sylitol.

## Unsweetened beverages

Beverages include tea, coffee, water, and sparkling water.

## Herbs and spices

These include black pepper, salt, basil, rosemary, curry, turmeric, cumin, cilantro, chives, dill, garlic, green onion, ginger, nutmeg, cinnamon, chili powder, thyme, parsley, paprika, and oregano.

## Miscellaneous items

These include capers, olives, mustard, balsamic vinegar, apple cider vinegar, white wine vinegar, rice vinegar, white vinegar, seaweed, miso paste, sauerkraut, nutritional yeast, kimchi, amino acids, red wine vinegar, baking soda, baking powder, and cornstarch.

If you choose to add a few animal-based products to your diet, here are a few guidelines:

- Poultry: choose free-range, organic sources.
- Dairy and eggs: use organic products obtained from animals raised in pastures.
- Seafood: obtain wild-caught sources from sustainable fisheries.
- Pork and beef: obtain grass-fed or pasture-raised sources.

## Foods to Use in Small Quantities

- Eggs
- Dairy

- Beef
- Pork
- Chicken
- Seafood
- Lamb
- Game meats

**Foods to Avoid**

- Processed foods like packaged foods (crackers, frozen dinners, chips, and cereal bars)
- Foods with added sugars like soda, candy, cereal with high sugar content, and cookies.
- Refined grains like white bread, white rice, and refined pasta.
- Fast foods like hot dogs, chicken nuggets, cheeseburgers, and fried chicken.
- Processed animal products like sausage, beef jerky, lunch meat, and bacon.
- Artificial sweeteners like Splenda and Equal.

# Benefits to Practicing a Plant-Based Diet

There are several health benefits to practicing a plant-based diet, and they include:

- Lowering the risk of unhealthy weight gain and overeating. People who practice a plant-based diet tend to feel full faster; therefore, they eat smaller portions. In addition, the calories they consume are burned quickly and cleanly. When practiced with an exercise regimen, a plant-based diet can help slim you down easily and without fuss.

- Lowering the risk of developing cardiovascular diseases, such as heart disease and stroke. Consuming fruits, vegetables, whole grains, nuts, seeds, and legumes provide the body with good cholesterol while lowering the levels of bad cholesterol, which is a major contributing factor to the development of poor cardiovascular health.
- Aids in decreasing inflammation within the body. Consuming raw plant-based foods that are rich in antioxidants and probiotics helps to decrease the symptoms of rheumatoid arthritis, which includes swelling, morning stiffness, and joint pain.
- Offers protection against certain types of cancer such as breast, colon, and prostate cancer. Consuming legumes on a regular basis, consuming soy-based products, and eliminating or minimizing the consumption of animal products helps in the risk reduction of developing these cancers.
- Allows the practitioner to consume high amounts of nutrients such as fiber, antioxidants, vitamins such as Vitamin C, Vitamin D, Vitamin K, Vitamin D and vitamin E, and minerals such as magnesium, folate, and potassium.

## How to Transition to a Plant-Based Diet

Starting a new diet can be hard and requires some planning, effort, and maybe even willpower. There are a few strategies that you can employ to make your transition to a plant-based diet easier:

- Know what your motivation for practicing a plant-based diet is. It may be that you want to eat healthier. It may also be that you want to leave a smaller environmental footprint as this is one of the benefits of practicing a plant-based diet. It may be because you want to enhance the medicinal benefits you gain from using herbal medicine. Whatever your motivation is, write it down and remind yourself regularly of why you have changed your diet.

- Stop slowly by picking a few plant-based meals and rotating them throughout the week. Oatmeal, stir-fried veggies, beans, and brown rice bowls and lentil soup are a great starting point. Another great option for starting slow is to switch up only one meal for the week, such as breakfast, to a plant-based option.

- Eat variety. Practicing a plant-based diet does not mean that you eat only carrots every day. With the thousands of options in fruit, veggies and whole grains available, you can switch it up every day so that your palette get something rewarding, and you do not get bored.

- Rid your kitchen cabinets of processed foods. It is easy to reach for something that is in easy reach, so cleaning out your cupboards of processed food makes it easier to transition to a plant-based diet. Instead, stock up your shelves and refrigerator with healthy, unprocessed, or minimally-processed foods.

- Ensuring that you have plant-based options to get in your daily recommended value of protein. By minimizing or avoiding proteins obtained from animal sources such as meat and eggs, you may come up with a deficit of protein in your diet. But you can quickly fill up this gap with plant-based protein options, such as chickpeas, nuts, seeds, legumes, tofu and tempeh.

- Keep on educating yourself about plant-based eating. Even in this age of technology, it is easy to become misinformed due to false information being published at the click of a finger. It is important that you keep yourself informed from reliable sources so that you can properly plan your plant-based diet.

- Surround yourself with like-minded people. Humans are social creatures and tend to be impacted by the crowd that they run with. It is easy to feel isolated if you are the only one practicing a plant-based diet in a crowd that consumes processed foods regularly. Therefore, to ensure that you do not yield to social pressure to revert to a diet of processed foods, it is a great idea to find like-minded people who practice a plant-based diet and medicine. You do not even need to leave your house to do this as social media has made it easy to find people with similar interests.

- Plan your meals. Having weekly meal plans are great for keeping you on track with your eating since they take the guesswork out of what you will eat daily. To help get you started, please find the sample 7-day meal plan below.

## 7-Day Plant-Based Meal Plan

### Day 1

Breakfast: Chickpea omelette

Lunch: Chickpea salad topped with fresh chopped veggies, avocado, and pumpkin seeds

Dinner: Zucchini curry

Snack 1: Kale chips

Snack 2: Carrot sticks dipped in roasted tahini veggie dip

## Day 2

Breakfast: Coconut milk oatmeal topped with coconut flakes, berries, and walnuts

Lunch: No-meat butternut squash chili

Dinner: Cauliflower rice stir-fry

Snack 1: Coconut chips

Snack 2: Parmesan popcorn

## Day 3

Breakfast: Chocolate banana pancakes

Lunch: Quinoa topped with veggies and feta

Dinner: Black bean and sweet potato tacos

Snack 1: Sweet potato chips

Snack 2: Celery sticks dipped in cashew butter

## Day 4

Breakfast: Almond banana granola served with coconut milk

Lunch: Hummus veggie wraps

Dinner: Gluten-free vegan macaroni and cheese

Snack 1: Tofu chips

Snack 2: Granola

## Day 5

Breakfast: Overnight oats topped with chia seeds and fresh berries

Lunch: Vegan BLT sandwich

Dinner: Grilled tempeh with roasted broccoli and potatoes

Snack 1: Trail mix

Snack 2: Fresh fruit like banana or pear slices

**Day 6**

Breakfast: Blueberry muffins

Lunch: Cauliflower and lentil curry

Dinner: Eggplant lasagna with green salad

Snack 1: Roasted chickpeas

Snack 2: Berry banana smoothie

**Day 7**

Breakfast: Kale blackberry smoothie with cashew butter and coconut milk

Lunch: Tahini quinoa and roasted veggies

Dinner: Black bean burgers

Snack 1: Dried figs

Snack 2: Apple slices dipped in peanut butter

# Chapter 8: Essentials Oils

It is common to hear essential oils and aromatherapy used in conjunction with each other, but many people do not understand the tremendous positive impact that both can have on their lives. This chapter is dedicated to explaining what are essential oils and their health benefits in addition to giving you a comprehensive list of the different types and the effects. It should be noted that essential oils do not work for everyone, yet some people swear by the medicinal effects it afforded them. There is no harm in trying them to see if they work for you.

## What are Essential Oils?

Essential oils are the resulting ingredient when compounds have been extracted from plants. They are so called because they capture the 'essence' or scent of the plant. Essential oils are created through the process of distillation, which uses steam or water or a mechanical methods like cold-pressing. Once the aromatic compounds have been extracted from the plant, they are combined with a carrier oil to create a final product.

A carrier oil is also created from a plant; however, it is used to dilute essential oils so that they can be carried on your skin. Essential oils are very potent and can cause irritation if they are applied directly to the skin. Examples of carrier oils include olive oil, black seed oil, avocado oil, sunflower oil, sweet almond oil, grapeseed oil, and coconut oil. They are unscented or lightly scented and do not interfere with the function of the essential oil. They are nourishing to skin. Essential oils are used by inhaling or applying topically to skin. They should never be swallowed.

## The History of Essential Oil Use

Essential oils and aromatherapy originated in Ancient Egypt. Egyptians cultivated plants to create oils that were used in cosmetic, medicinal, and religious purposes. These oils were also used for embalming.

These oils were extracted through a solvent extraction method using animal fat in the early stage of the use of essential oils. However, there is evidence that the distillation process has been used since 3500 BC.

It was not long after, Indian and Chinese cultures started exploring the use of aromatherapy. The practices of the Egyptians were adopted by the Greeks around 400 BC. It was introduced by well-known physician Hippocrates, who was a firm believer of using holistic practices to treat patients. This knowledge was then adopted by the Romans to promote good health. Aromatic baths were especially popular at that time.

The use of essential oils went through a dark period after the fall of the Roman Empire. It was repressed by religious denominations that considered bathing a sin. The use of aromatics to cover stench was practiced, and the practices that Hippocrates encouraged were forgotten.

Luckily, there was a rebirth of interest in aromatherapy and essential oil usage in the Renaissance period. A physician called Paracelsus (1493-1541) helped with this introduction by claiming to "cure leprosy" with the use of plant extracts. The term aromatherapy was then invented by a French chemist and perfumer called Rene Maurice Gattefosse in 1937.

Interest in aromatherapy exploded in the late 70s and early 80s due to a boom in interest in natural medicine.

## What is Aromatherapy?

Aromatherapy is also called essential oil therapy. It is a holistic approach to promoting good health and wellness through the use of natural plant extracts. These essential oils improve health mentally, physically, and emotionally through the medicinal properties of these oils. Essential oil therapy has been used by humans for thousands of years and was popular in ancient cultures, such as Egyptian, Indian and Chinese. Its benefits can still be gained today.

### *Benefits of Aromatherapy and Essential Oils*

- Helps improve digestion
- Aids in pain management
- Improves sleep quality and helps fight insomnia
- Soothes sore joints
- Treats migraines and headaches
- Aids in easing the discomfort of child labor
- Helps alleviate the side effects of chemotherapy
- Reduces inflammation
- Reduces stress and anxiety
- Aids in the treatment of asthma
- Helps reduce PMS and menopausal symptoms
- Aids in reducing the symptoms of arthritis
- Aids in treating erectile dysfunction
- Can be used an antibiotic and antimicrobial agent

Aromatherapy affords these benefits through the smell of and the skin absorption of the essential oils. Aromatherapy works by using the following products, which can be used in combination or alone:

- Inhalers
- Diffusers
- Aroma spritzers
- Body oils, lotions, and creams
- Facial steamers
- Clay masks
- Hot and cold compresses
- Bath salts

## How Essential Oils Work

When essential oils are inhaled, they stimulate specific areas in the limbic system. The limbic system is a part of the brain where emotions, long-term memory, sense of smell, and behavior are controlled. It is interesting that this part of the brain aids in forming memories and regulating emotions as it explains why certain smells trigger memories or emotions in some people.

The limbic system also helps to control some unconscious bodily functions, such as heart rate, blood pressure and breathing. The use of essential oils has been reported to enhance or help regulate some of these functions by some users.

When essential oils are applied to the skin, they are absorbed to interact with the body in a variety of ways.

## Other Uses of Essential Oils

In addition to be used in aromatherapy, essential oils have the following uses:

- To freshen up the scent of homes, cars, and offices
- To freshen up the scent of laundry
- As an insect repellent
- To add a natural scent to homemade cosmetics
- To extend the shelf-life of some foods

## Types of Essential Oils and the Part of the Plant That They Are Derived From

Essential oils can be derived from one part of a plant or several parts of the plant.

### *Derived from the leaves*

- Bay laurel
- Bergamot mint
- Cajeput
- Cinnamon
- Eucalyptus
- Geranium
- Lemon Myrtle
- Myrtle
- Niaouli
- Ravensara
- Tea tree
- Tobacco

- Violet

**Derived from the flowers**

- Boronia
- Chamomile
- Clove
- Diwana
- Jasmine
- Lindale blossom
- Rose
- Tuberose
- Ylang ylang

**Derived from flowering herbs**

The oils are created through the distillation of both the flowers and the leaves. They include:

- Basil
- Catnip
- Holy basil
- Hyssop
- Lavender
- Lavandin
- Lemon balm
- Marjoram
- Oregano
- Peppermint
- Rosemary

- Sage
- Spearmint
- Thyme
- Yarrow

***Derived from the bark***

- Cassia
- Cinnamon

***Derived from the wood***

- Amyris
- Cedarwood
- Palo Santo
- Rosewood
- Sandalwood

***Derived from the needles***

- Cypress
- Fir
- Scotch pine
- Spruce

***Derived from the grass***

- Citronella
- Lemongrass
- Palmarosa

***Derived from citrus rinds***

- Bergamot

- Grapefruit
- Lemon
- Lime
- Mandarin
- Orange
- Tangerine

***Derived from the gum, resin, or balsam***

- Benzoin
- Peru balsam
- Elemi
- Galbanum
- Gurjum

***Derived from berries or fruit***

- Allspice
- Black pepper
- Juniper berry
- May Chang

***Derived from moss or lichen***

- Oak moss

***Derived from Roots***

- Angelica
- Ginger
- Vetiver

***Derived from seeds***

- Ambrette
- Anise
- Cardamom
- Carrot
- Coffee bean
- Coriander
- Cumin
- Dill
- Fennel
- Nutmeg
- Parsley

# Popular Essential Oils and Their Health Benefits

- Angelica root. This helps support a healthy immune and respiratory system in addition to fighting stress, fatigue, and tension. It also aids in restoring strength and stamina.
- Bergamot. This helps reduce stress and improve certain skin conditions like eczema.
- Black pepper. The spicy scent aids in soothing muscle aches, supports a healthy digestive system, and stimulates appetite.
- Cajeput. This aids in treating skin conditions like insect bites, blemishes, and excess oil production. It also aids in relieving minor joint and muscle pain.

- Chamomile. Best essential oil aids in improving mood and promoting relaxation.
- Citronella. This is a mosquito repellent.
- Eucalyptus. This essential oil aids in clearing congestion and is an anti-inflammatory.
- Geranium. This helps relieve hormonal headaches.
- Jasmine. This is in alleviating the pains of childbirth, enhances libido, and fights depression.
- Lavender. It aids in relieving stress and helps soothe allergy-related symptoms. It is also an anti-inflammatory agent and helps relieve migraines.
- Lemon. Lemon oil helps improve mood, treats headaches, and improve digestion.
- Peppermint. Aids in digestion and boosts energy. It is also an anti-inflammatory and helps relieve tension headaches.
- Rose. This is essential oil is in reducing anxiety and improving mood.
- Sandalwood. This essential oil is improving focus and concentration in addition to calming nerves. It also helps relieve the symptoms of allergies, such as runny nose and sneezing.
- Ylang ylang. This is in the treatment of certain skin conditions, nausea, and headaches.

## The Dangers of Improper Usage of Essential oils

The benefits that essential oils can afford are numerous and far-reaching. However, if essential oils are used incorrectly, they can cause poisoning even if small amounts are ingested.

Essential oils are not fit for consumption and should always be diluted with carrier oils to decrease the potency. If this is not done, allergic reactions, skin rashes and burns are possible. Children are especially susceptible. The severity of the toxicity that an essential oil has depends on the type of oil and the amount that has been ingested. Symptoms of toxicity include:

- Seizures
- Persistent coughing
- Nausea
- Vomiting
- Diarrhea
- Skin irritation
- Redness, irritation, or pain in the eyes
- Drowsiness
- Shallow breathing
- Coma in cases where a large amount has been ingested

Luckily, there are steps you can take to minimize the damage in case of exposure. If the essential oil has been swallowed, rinse out the mouth and call your local poison information center. Do not intake any oral fluids until that is advised by the local poison information center. Ingesting fluids can cause aspiration of fluid into the lungs or vomiting, which should not be induced.

If eye exposure to essential oil occurs, immediately rinse out the eyes using running water. Allow the flowing water to run from the corner of the eye closest to the nose over the eye and outward. They should be done for 15 minutes, and the eye should be evaluated by a licensed medical doctor.

If excessive inhalation of essential oil occurs, the affected person should be taken into an open area where they can breathe in fresh air. If this does not help in settling the symptoms, the local poison information center should be called.

If pure essential oil is exposed to the skin, then the skin should be washed with clean water and soap after all contaminated clothing has been removed. If the symptoms are not resolved by this, a licensed medical doctor should be seen.

Essential oils should be handled with caution and only after they have been properly diluted with carrier oils. Extra caution should be taken when essential oils are handled by pregnant and breastfeeding women and children.

# The Do's and Don'ts of Using Essential Oil Safely

### The Do's

When purchasing essential oils, check the quality to ensure that any extra ingredients added are not detrimental to your health. Not all added ingredients are bad, so you simply need to be vigilant.

Test a small bit of the essential oil on a small part of your arm or leg before using large amounts. This will allow you to see how you skin responds. Some people have had skin irritation and an allergic reaction to using essential oils.

Stop the use of essential oil immediately if you notice undesirable skin reactions, such as rashes, itchiness, and little bumps. This applies even if the essential oil is an ingredient in another produce like a cream. Wash the product off with soap and clean water.

Store essential oils correctly. They should be kept at room temperature in a dry area that is out of reach of young children.

### *The Don'ts*

Do not rub essential oils on your body indiscriminately. They are not safe to put in your nose, eyes, mouth, or private areas. The arms and legs are safe application areas.

Do not apply essential oils to damaged skin. This doubly applies to undiluted essential oils. The application of essential oils to inflamed or injured skin can cause adverse skin reactions.

Do not keep or use essential oils that are more than three years old. Past this point the essential oil would have likely spoiled due to oxygen exposure. Not only do the essential oils do not work as well, but they can cause allergies reaction or skin irritation. If you notice that your essential oil had changed in color, texture or smell, throw it out and replace it.

Do not overuse essential oil. The old adage that too much of a good thing is bad. Even when essential oils are diluted, they can cause a negative reaction when used too often or in amounts that are too large.

# Chapter 9: Herbal Medicine

## What are Medicinal Plants?

These are also referred to as medicinal herbs and have been used for illness prevention and cure since historic times. These are handy plants to keep around to treat common ailments, such as tummy aches, headaches, and even the symptoms of bug bites. They can be used in teas, as food garnishes, inhalants, and applied topically. This chapter is dedicated to providing you with a long list of medicinal plants that are great to keep around your home to keep your body in tip-top shape the natural way.

### *Common Medicinal Plants and their Health Benefits*

**Thyme**

Thyme is popular for use in cooking, but not many people know about its medicinal functions. Thyme health benefits include:

- Treating respiratory issues
- Supporting a healthy immune system
- Improving blood circulation
- Soothing sore throats and coughs

These benefits are made possible because of the presence of the compound called thymol in the plant. This compound has antifungal and antibacterial properties. These properties help in preventing foodborne diseases by decontaminating food and preventing infections from occurring in the body. Due to these properties, thymol is a common ingredient in vapor rubs and mouthwash. To benefit from thyme, you can brew its leaves for tea, use as a garnish for meals, or apply topically as a cream.

## Kava Kava

Kava kava goes by the scientific name of Piper methysticum. The name kava means bitter. The plant has been used by Pacific Islanders for thousands of years to:

- Reduce pain
- Reduce the risk of cancer
- Protect neurons from damage
- Reduce anxiety
- As a sleep aid

Kava kava is most often brewed as a tea.

## Echinacea

This is an herbaceous flowering plant from the daisy family that is found in Eastern and Central North America. It mainly grows in prairies and open wooded areas. This plant activates a chemical in the body that helps fight the symptoms of the cold and flu by decreasing inflammation in the body. In addition to fighting the common, echinacea also:

- Increases athletic performance
- Fights gingivitis
- Decreases anxiety
- Prevents the formation of anal warts that are caused by the human papilloma virus (HPV)
- Aids in treating indigestion
- Aids in treating yeast
- Acts as a pain reliever

- Fights migraine headaches
- Fights indigestion

## Sage

The official name of this plant is salvia officinalis. Sage is well known in the diabetic community for its ability to naturally lowering glucose levels. It also helps support memory and combats degenerative diseases. Sage can be used to prepare dishes as well as in beauty products. It's health benefits include:

- Supporting digestive health
- Strengthening the immune system
- Aiding in the treatment and management of diabetes
- Improving skin health
- Improving memory
- Enhancing overall brain function
- Supplying antioxidants

You can reap these benefits by brewing the fresh leaves for tea, inhaling it as an essential oil, applying the essential oil topically, and using as a garnish for meals.

## Rosemary

The official name of this medicinal plant is Rosmarinus officinalis. Rosemary is filled with essential vitamins and minerals that help to support the function of a healthy body in addition to medicinal benefits. Its medicinal benefits include:

- Supporting a healthy liver
- Support health hair growth
- Reducing inflammation
- Treating halitosis

- Improving memory
- Enhancing overall brain function
- Improving blood circulation

Gain these benefits by brewing the dried leaves for tea, applying the essential oil topically and using as a garnish for meals.

**Parsley**

Parsley, also known as petroselinum crispum, is known as a delicious garnish in the cooking world, but did you know that it helps support several of the body's essential systems such as the immune system? Because of it's high concentration of Vitamin K and antioxidants, it also aids in boosting overall body health. Parsley's health benefits include:

- Fighting halitosis
- Supporting bone health
- Relieving bloating
- Supporting digestive health
- Supplying antioxidants

In addition to using this as a garnish in dishes, it can be used to brew tea and create juices.

**Peppermint**

This herb is commonly found in toothpaste, gum and even in deserts, but its health benefits are numerous. They include:

- Treating halitosis
- Supporting digestive health
- As an antibacterial agent
- Relieving digestive issues such as gas indigestion and nausea

- Relieving headaches
- Soothing muscle pain
- Relieving allergies

These benefits can be obtained by brewing the leaves in tea, inhaling the essential oil, and applying the essential oil topically.

## Basil

The scientific name of Basil is ocimum basilicum. It is commonly used to add flavor to the dishes and as a garnish. Basil is rich in vitamins and minerals such as vitamin k and iron. This rich nutritional value helps combat common ailments. Basil's many health benefits include:

- Aiding in the metabolism of different compounds in the body
- Acting as an antibacterial agent
- Supplying the body with antioxidants
- Boosting immunity
- Improving digestion
- Strengthening bone and liver health
- Reducing inflammation
- Slowing the aging process
- Reducing stress

In addition to using basil as a garnish, it can be used as an ingredient to create smoothies.

## Catnip

The scientific name for catnip is nepeta cataria. Most people are familiar with catnip's role in attracting cats to roll around in it. This is because it is a stimulant for the animals. It also acts as a sedative if the cat consumes it. It has a variety of effects on humans, including being a sleep aid and a stress reliever. These effects come from the presence of compounds such as thymol and nepetalactone. The health benefits of catnip include:

- Reducing anxiety and stress
- Inducing calmness
- Accelerating the recovery from fevers and colds
- Relieving stomach aches
- Acting as a bug repellent
- Relieving skin irritation from bug bites

People can reap the benefits of catnip by brewing its leaves in tea, drying the leaves and burning to release the aroma and applying the leaves or essential oil topically.

**Chamomile**

Scientifically referred to as matricaria chamomilla, chamomile is great at relieving a variety of illnesses and elements because of his high concentration of antioxidants. Many people are familiar with chamomile as tea and use it to relax just before bed. Its other health benefits include:

- Relieving pain
- Reducing inflammation
- Relieving congestion
- Improving skin health
- Acting as a sleep aid

Chamomile can be used by brewing the dry leaves, inhaling as an essential oil, and applying topically.

## Cayenne Pepper

Best known for adding a spicy kick to a meal or drink, cayenne pepper goes by the scientific name of capsicum annuum. The main compound responsible for cayenne pepper's role as a medicinal plant is called capsaicin. It is responsible for the spicy nature of cayenne pepper but also the health benefits that include:

- Relieving pain
- Lowering cholesterol
- Improving blood circulation
- Easing upset stomach
- Aiding in digestion
- Boosting metabolism
- Detoxifying the body

While cayenne pepper can be consumed as a pill, it is commonly added to dressings, spice mixes, sauces, and other dishes.

## Dandelion

This plant goes by the scientific name of taraxacum. While it is known as a pesky weed, you may want to think twice before you pluck it out of your front yard. Many people do not know this, but the dandelion is edible and full of health benefits because of its high nutritional value that includes Vitamin C, Vitamin K, calcium, iron, and more. Even the dandelion root affords a person many great health benefits, which include:

- Improving skin health
- Treating skin infections
- Supporting bone health

- Treating and preventing urinary tract infections
- Detoxifying the liver
- Supporting liver health

Dandelion roots can be brewed as a tea and its leaves can be used as a garnish for dishes.

## Garlic

Garlic goes by the scientific name of allium sativum and is considered a super-plant for fighting infections and aiding in the improvement of overall health. The health benefits of garlic include:

- Lowering cholesterol and blood pressure
- Aiding preventing the development of degenerative diseases such as Alzheimer's and dementia
- Improve in digestive health
- Preventing the development of cardiovascular diseases such as heart disease
- Boosting the function of the immune system

Garlic can be consumed raw, cooked as an ingredient in dishes and used to garnish dishes.

## Marigold

Going by the scientific name of tagetes, this medicine of plant is known for its fragrant nature. It is chock-full of antioxidants and other health-boosts in compounds that make it a great choice to keep around your home. Its benefits include:

- Treating skin diseases
- Soothing skin infections
- Boosting eye health
- As an antibacterial and antiseptic agent

- Reducing inflammation
- Treating eye pain and infection

A person can gain these health benefits from marigold by brewing the dried flowers for tea, using as a garnish in dishes, or applying the essential oil or cream topically.

**Lemon Balm**

Known scientifically as Melissa officinalis, this must be Santa plant is delicious and contains a variety of compounds that aid in:

- Reducing anxiety and stress
- Soothing menstrual cramps
- Reducing inflammation
- Treating cold sores
- Soothing restless children

To gain these health benefits you know how lemon balm's leaves can be brewed as a tea, applied topically as an essential oil, or used to garnish dishes and desserts.

**Tulsi**

This is an aromatic perennial plant that goes by the scientific name of ocimum tenuiflorum. This plant is also called holy basil and is celebrated for its remarkable holistic healing properties. These remedies include:

- Providing protection against insect bites and bacteria
- Providing relief from colds, bronchitis, coughs, and fever
- Relief against indigestion
- Aids in curing malaria
- Headache relief

This plant can be brewed as a tea and used to make an essential oil. It is commonly used in ayurveda medicine and comes in four varieties. This plant is native to India and is widespread across the Southeast Asian tropics.

**Aloe vera**

Aloe vera is a plant that is grown in tropical climates all around the world and is native to North America, Southern Europe, and the Canary islands. There are even records of its medicinal use dating back to ancient Egypt. This plant has a variety of medicinal uses including:

- Providing relief against sunburn
- Healing wounds
- Relieving heartburn
- Reducing inflammation
- Help slow the spread of breast cancer
- Can be used to maintain oral health
- Aids lowering blood sugar levels
- Works as a natural laxative
- Used to grow fuller, longer hair
- Helps fight acne breakouts

Aloe vera has over 500 species. The succulent plant is stemless.

**Ashwagandha**

Translated in skerritt, ashwagandha means "smell of a horse." This meaning references the plants unique smell and its ability to increase body strength. The scientific name is withania somnifera, but it also goes by other names, including winter cherry and the Indian ginseng. The proven health benefits of this plant include:

- Fighting inflammation
- Fighting tumor growth
- Lowering blood sugar levels
- Lowering cortisol levels. Cortisol is a stress hormone that is released from the adrenal glands in response to stress and when blood sugar levels are too low. The release of cortisol can become a chronic problem if it is uncontrolled and has detrimental health effects.
- Aids in reducing anxiety and stress
- Helps boost testosterone levels
- Aids an increasing fertility in men
- Aids in increasing muscle mass and body strength

## Stevia

In addition to being a natural sweetener, stevia has a host of medical uses. They include:

- Fighting cavities other oral problems
- Helping to control blood sugar levels
- Aids in fighting type 2 diabetes
- Helping to control weight gain
- Helping to lower blood pressure
- Helping to strengthen bones
- Aids in preventing upper respiratory infections.

Stevia is a perennial shrub that belongs to the sunflower family. It is indigenous to South America and has over 200 species. The compounds that gives stevia leaf its sweet taste are called stevioside and rebaudioside A. These compounds were isolated in 1931, but it was during World War II that stevia was promoted as an alternative to sugar when sugar was in short supply. Stevia was used by Japanese in the 1970s to replace the banned artificial sweetener called saccharine.

**Marsh mellow**

As the name suggests this is the plant from which marshmallows were once made from. However, apart from its use in the confectionery treat, the roots and leaves of this plant we used to treat aching muscles, bruises, insect bites, gastritis, inflammation of the urinary and respiratory mucous membranes, as a counter to excessive stomach acid production, and to treat bruises and sprains. The leaves of this plant are edible and can be fried, boiled, or added to salads.

# Probiotics

Probiotics are live yeast and bacteria that reside in your body and are good for you. They are especially prominent in your digestive system. Typically, when people think of bacteria, they think of disease and infection, but the body is filled with bacteria that aid in upkeeping health because they help keep your gut healthy. While the body does indeed contains bad bacteria, good gut health depends on keeping a balance of the good and bad bacteria.

*Types of Probiotics*

- Lactobacillus. This is the type of probiotic that comes to mind when most people think of probiotic. It is commonly found in fermented foods and yogurt and can help people who are lactose intolerant. Different strains of lactobacillus can help stop diarrhea.

- Bifidobacterium. This type of probiotic is typically found in dairy products and can be used to ease the symptoms of irritable bowel syndrome (IBS) among several other conditions.

- Saccharomyces boulardii. This is a yeast. It helps fight diarrhea and other digestive issues.

## Benefits of Probiotics

Eating a variety of probiotic rich foods gains a person the following benefits:

- Reduced risk of developing cancer. Scientific research has shown that the disturbance of the balance between good bacteria and bad bacteria in the gut can cause the uncontrolled development of cells, which can lead to cancer. Promoting the balance of bacteria in the gut reduces this risk.

- Reduced the risk of developing inflammatory bowel disease (IBD). This too is a condition that depends on the balance of good and bad bacteria in the gut. Keeping the balance tipped on the side of probiotics aids in lowering the risk of developing the condition.

- Improved digestion. Probiotics speed up the digestion process by breaking down food faster so that it does not linger in the digestive system. The aid that probiotics provide reduces the risk of developing symptoms of Crohn's disease, irritable bowel syndrome (IBS), and constipation.

- Aid in diabetes management. Probiotics improve glycemic control and lipid metabolism in persons with type 2 diabetes.

- Reduced risk of developing metabolic diseases. Metabolic diseases include type 2 diabetes, liver disease, and obesity. The regular consumption of probiotics can prevent and aid in the management of these conditions.

- The maintenance of vaginal health. The vagina contains several bacteria and spermicides and contraceptives, and antibiotics can throw off the delicate balance that ensures good health of the tract. This can cause infection. Regular consumption of probiotics can restore the balance and prevent infections and other issues.

- Help in maintaining mental health. The health of your gut can influence your mental health. Therefore, a regular consumption of probiotics can reduce the symptoms of mental disorders such as anxiety and depression.
- Reduces side effects from antibiotics. More than 30% of people who take antibiotics develop the side effect of antibiotic-associated diarrhea. Taking probiotics alongside antibiotics can prevent the development of the side effects.

## *Plant-Based Probiotics*

While yogurt is one of the most popular sources of probiotics, there are plant-based options available. See below for just a few of these.

### Sauerkraut

This is simply fermented cabbage. It is created by finely cutting up cabbage and fermenting it in brine, which is a concentrate of salt water. It is rich in vitamin C, vitamin K and potassium, in addition to the probiotic, lactobacillus.

### Kimchi

This is also another fermented cabbage dish and only differs from sauerkraut through the addition of spices and a few vegetables. It is rich in vitamins, antioxidants, and the same type of probiotic as sauerkraut.

## Miso

This is a Japanese seasoning made from soybeans, fermented salt, and a fungus called koji. In addition to its probiotic health benefits, it helps lower the risk of developing breast cancer and having a stroke. It is rich in various nutritional components such as protein, fiber, vitamins, and minerals.

## Tempeh

This is a fermented soybean product that originated in Indonesia but is popular worldwide as a high-protein meat substitute. It is greatly used in vegan and vegetarian cooking.

## Pickles

Pickles are a vegetable that have been fermented in a brine solution. This fermenting process creates a probiotic-rich food. Almost any vegetable can be pickled, but some popular options include carrots, cucumbers, green beans, red bell peppers and cauliflower. These should be enjoyed in moderation because of their high sodium content, which can cause high blood pressure and water retention. To add extra flavor to pickles, herbs and spices, such as garlic, bay leaf, and coriander seeds can be added.

# List of Herbal Remedies

Below you will find a comprehensive list listed from A to Z of remedies and medicines that can prevent and treat everyday maladies and more serious conditions such as arthritis.

- Alfalfa. This can be used to lower cholesterol, in addition to treating kidney and urinary tract ailments.
- Aloe vera. This can be used to treat skin infections and heal burns and wounds.
- Barberry. Barberry can be used to treat gastrointestinal disorders and skin infections.

- Bilberry. This aids in improving blood circulation and repairs blood veins.
- Bitter orange. This is used to treat allergic inflammation.
- Blueberries. In addition to being a powerful antioxidants, they can be used to treat urinary tract infections.
- Cat's claw. This is used to treat gastrointestinal disorder, to boost the immune system and as an anti-inflammatory agent.
- Celery. This can be used as a diuretic.
- Chaste berry. This is used to treat PMS and menopausal symptoms and acne.
- Cilantro. Aids in detoxifying the body and in digestion.
- Clove. This can be ingested to treat an upset stomach and applied topically to treat toothaches.
- Cranberry. This aids in treating urinary tract infections.
- Daisy. These can be ingested as a tea, and the leaves can be used in a salad. It can be used to treat respiratory tract and gastrointestinal disorders.
- Devil's claw. This is used to treat back pain, joint inflammation, and arthritis.
- Dong Quai. This is used to treat the symptoms of PMS and menopause in addition to treating migraines and cardiovascular problems.
- Echinacea. The purple flowers of this plant aids in treating the common cold, helps to boost immunity, and treats bronchitis and upper respiratory infections.

- Evening primrose. This helps relieve the symptoms of PMS and menopause. It also aids in treating mild skin conditions such as eczema, helps to regulate blood pressure and is an anti-inflammatory.

- Eucalyptus. This can be used as an analgesic and to treat coughs and colds.

- Fenugreek. This can be used to treat the symptoms of menopause in addition to digestive issues and loss of appetite.

- Feverfew. Just as the name suggests, the leaves of this plant are used to treat fevers in addition to treating migraines and arthritis.

- Flaxseed. This is an anti-inflammatory, aids in weight loss management, aids in regulating blood pressure, and helps prevent colon cancer.

- Ginger. This aids in treating motion sickness and nausea.

- Gingko. This plant helps boost brain health and treats degenerative diseases like mild to moderate dementia and Alzheimer's disease. It also aids in treating mental illnesses, such as depression and anxiety and improving eye health.

- Ginseng. This can be used as an aphrodisiac and as a tonic to enhance vitality.

- Goldenseal. This is used to treat diarrhea, skin infections, and eye irritations. It can also be used as an antiseptic.

- Grape seed extract. This aids in lowering bad (LDL) cholesterol, regulating blood pressure, reducing the symptoms of poor circulation in leg veins, and is an anti-cancer agent.

- Green tea. The leaves of these can be used as a tonic to improve overall health and as an antioxidant.
- Guarana. This plant can be used as a tonic, to treat diarrhoea and control appetite.
- Guava. It can be used to treat diarrhea.
- Henna. This is an antibacterial and anti-inflammatory agent that has analgesic properties
- Horsetail. This can be used to treat tuberculosis and kidney problems in addition to healing wounds and ulcers and stopping bleeding.
- Jasmine. This is an anti-inflammatory and antiseptic agent.
- Lemon. The resulting liquid from combining the juice of this plant with honey can be used to treat sore throats and coughs.
- Milk thistle. The fruit of this plant is used to treat high cholesterol and liver condition in addition to reducing the growth of cancer cells.
- Mullein. Commonly added to cough syrups, this plant helps heal bronchial respiratory infections.
- Oregano. This can be used to treat stomach and respiratory ailments.
- Papaya. This can be used to treat stomach aches and wounds.
- Plantain. The leaves of this plant can be brewed in a tea, which can be used to fight coughs. The leaves can also be applied topically to treat skin infections and insect bites.

- Saint John's wort. The leaf and flower of this plant can be used as an antidepressant.
- Saw palmetto. The fruit of this plant can be used to treat benign prostatic hypertrophy.
- Star anise. This can be used to treat influenza.
- Tea tree oil. This oil is derived from the leaves of a tree that is native to Australia. It is beneficial in treating acne, dandruff, insect bites, and athlete's foot.
- Turmeric. This is an anti-inflammatory and aids in treating arthritis and skin diseases. It also aids in stopping the DNA mutations and helps prevent cancer.
- Valerian. The roots of this plant can be used to treat anxiety and as a sleep aid.
- Watercress. This can be used as an antibacterial agent and as a diuretic.
- Wild yam. This can be used to treat the symptoms of PMS and menopause in addition to being an anti-inflammatory agent. It also aids in relaxing muscles.

# Chapter 10: Medicinal Garden

You do not have to have a green thumb to grow an amazing medicinal herb and spice garden. This section is dedicated to showing you some of the easiest plants to grow and how you can maintain this garden no matter the amount of space that you have at your disposal. To relief from diarrhea and migraines and many other health issues, you can have them all by just stepping outside of your door. Keep reading to learn more.

## Benefits of Planting Your Own Medicinal Garden

There are several benefits to growing your own medicinal spice and herb garden. They include:

- Having more control over what you put into your body. Even though you pick up herbs and spices on your market or grocery store shelf, you have no way of truly knowing how these were grown and what chemicals that were used to assist the growth and maintenance process even if they claim to be organic. Chemicals like fertilizers can leave trace amounts on the plants, and these amounts can be ingested when we eat them. No matter how small these amounts are, they can burden us with dangerous their side effects and negative health consequences. By growing your own garden, you can have the security of knowing it is truly organic.
- Saving money. Often, all you need to get started with your own herb and spice garden is a packet of seeds. These cost next to nothing and keep on giving since the

plants produce their own seeds most times. In addition, using these organic plants save you thousands of dollars in doctor's visits and bills every year when the resulting plants are used medicinally and in eating.

- Having a positive environmental impact. Gardens of all types attract insects like bees, butterflies and birds because they live off of the plants and the other types of creatures they attract. Birds and bees are pollinators and aid in ensuring more plants grow for the greater good of the earth.

- Gardening is good for your health. There are the obvious health benefits of eating organic plants from your own garden, like getting a greater variety of vitamins and minerals and lowering the risk of developing certain diseases. However, there are other health benefits, such as doing more physical activity that helps to keep your heart strong and taking in fresh air, which aids in purifying the lungs. There is also the mental health benefit of aiding in fighting mental diseases, such as depression.

- Gardening allows you to feel more self-reliant. When you have your own garden, you are not reliant on the supply from supermarkets or big corporations that make the big bucks off of your need to eat and to have good health. This aids in boosting your sense of independence and self-sufficiency.

- Gardening makes your yard more beautiful. Fruits, vegetables, flowers, herbs, and spices come in all sizes, shapes, and colors. These variations help to break up the monotonous nature of concrete jungles. The variety brings vivacity to the landscape and makes the scenery more interesting to look at. These plants also bring life ad beauty inside homes and offices.

- Garden helps bring you back to your indigenous roots. There is something about turning soil and planting seeds that makes a person feel more connected with the earth and to our ancestors who used to garden, not out of convenience, but out of necessity for medicine and food.

# Planning Your Garden

The reason most gardens fail is not because the person does not have a green thumb or because the process is particularly tricky. It is because these people begin to garden without any garden knowledge or planning. Here are some of the considerations you need to make to ensure that your medicinal garden flourishes:

- Your climate
- The location
- Choosing the right herbs and spices for your garden
- After care of your plants and herbs and spices

### *The Types of Herbs and Spices That Should Be Planted in Different Climates*

Before you tried to plant any herb or spice in your garden, you need to ensure that the temperature range of the climate that you live in is suitable for growing that particular plant. A little research on the Internet or speaking with your local nursery can help you with this. Summer and tropical climates are great for growing most plants. However, winter type climates are less forgiving.

### Plants That Grow Well in Warm and Hot Climates

All of the burbs and spices that will be listed below require that the soil be well-drained and need to be attended to when conditions are soggy. Some plants need to be planted at the required distance apart so that they are not crowded and air circulation is not compromised.

The following plants need at least four hours of bright sunlight per day and thrive in morning sunlight. They include parsley, peppermint, rosemary, sage, tarragon, mint, oregano, cilantro, basil, and chives.

These plants need between six and eight hours of direct sunlight daily. They include dill, fennel, yarrow, licorice, lavender, and winter savory.

**Plants That Grow Well in Cold Climates**

While winter has fewer hours of sunlight and the chilling temperature can make it harder to grow herbs and spices, it is not impossible to do especially if you have an indoor garden or if you can temporarily house the plants inside. Many of the herbs and spices listed can be grown year-round as long as the proper care and precaution is taken to ensure that they still thrive during the winter months. Some of them go dormant in the winter months and come back with new growth in the spring.

To prepare these plants for winter, prune them a few weeks before the first frost of the fall season by removing any wooden or dead stems and snipping off the upper leaves. This will ensure that your plant has a better chance of surviving from winter to spring.

You can still use some of these plants throughout the winter by digging them up and transferring them to containers that will be kept indoors by a sunny window throughout the winter. Out of some of the herbs and spices listed above that grow great in warm and hot climates, there are a few that can also survive the winter weather as long as they are kept indoors next to a sunny window. They include oregano, sage, mint, chives, and thyme. On the other hand, there are herbs and spices that are well adapted to growing in cold weather and they include tarragon, lemon balm, catnip, parsley, horseradish, sorrel, and caraway.

## *Choosing the Right Location*

When choosing a location to grow your medicinal garden, the two factors you need to consider are how well lit the area is by sunlight and the availability of well-drained soil. Therefore, you can grow your medicinal garden if you have acres of yard space available or even if you live in a tiny apartment.

No matter what location you choose or have available for your garden, here are a few tips to get you started, especially if this is your first time trying your hand at gardening:

- Start small. This tip is especially useful if you live in an apartment or do not have much space for a garden. If you have yard space available, cultivate your plants in a few feet of space to see how it goes. If you live in an apartment, get one or two small pots. Herbs and spices like basil, chives, geranium, thyme, parsley, mint, bay laurel, and rosemary are great for planting in small spaces or in an apartment.

- Focus on growing a few different plants to begin with. Do not overdo it or try to grow every herb or spice that you can think of. Start with herbs and spices that you already use regularly and are relatively easy to grow.

- Choose an area that receives adequate sunlight or is lit by natural light bulbs to place your potted plants or to cultivate your yard space.

- Research the plants that you plan to plant so that you know that the conditions it thrives and avoid placing it under conditions that will destroy it.

- Use good soil to get started. Different plants need different types of soil to grow. Usually herbs and spices grow best in typical garden soil because it has good drainage. Most herbs and spices do not do well in sandy soil or heavy clay so adding compost can be a good option if these are the types of soil that you have available. Compost provides the soil with needed nutrition to help plants grow.

- Get a few worms. Worms do a great job at breaking down the organics in soil, which makes them easier for plants to absorb. Worms can usually be purchased at bait and tackle shops.

- Set a watering schedule for your plants. Some plants need to be watered more often than others. Over-watering can damage a plant as can under-watering. Research will tell you how much your plants need to be watered so that you can set up a proper schedule to keep the plants properly hydrated.

- Learn how to weed. Luckily, this is not a concern if you live in an apartment, but if you have yard space then you need to set up a schedule for this as well.

- Keep it interesting. As you get your footing with gardening, gradually add new plants to your collection and have fun with it.

# 9 Common Herbs and Spices That You Can Grow on Your Own

*Rosemary*

Rosemary is an evergreen shrub that produces blue flowers and has needle-like leaves. The scientific name of rosemary is rosmarinus officinalis. This scientific name translates into "mists of the seas" because of its gray-green color, which resembles the mist against the cliff of the seaside of the Mediterranean, where the plant originates.

The health benefits of rosemary include levels of antioxidants, acting as an anti-inflammatory, improving digestion, preventing brain aging, lowering the risk of developing certain cancers, and enhancing memory and concentration.

Rosemary is not a plant that is complicated to care for. All it needs is well-drained, sandy soil and between six and eight hours of sunlight. It thrives in warm, humid environments and cannot withstand temperatures below 50 degrees Fahrenheit. Therefore, it needs to be transplanted from the soil to a container during winter months and kept indoors near a sunny window.

Rosemary plants are usually grown via the cuttings because the seeds are tricky to germinate. In fact, the seeds only germinate when they are very fresh and planted in conditions that are optimum. To propagate rosemary plants using cuttings, cut a two-inch stem from an existing to rosemary plant and remove the leaves on the bottom two-thirds of the way down of the cutting. Place this cutting in a mixture of peat moss and pertile. Spray the cutting with water. Once the roots have developed, the plants should successfully grow. Rosemary plants should be repotted at least once every year because they have a tendency to become root bound, which is the condition that causes a plant's roots to fill its container, leaving no more room for the plant to expand. Luckily, the yellowing of the plant will indicate that it is time to repot.

## *Parsley*

Parsley comes from the same family as dill and has bright green, feather-like leaves. It is a biennial plant, which means that it takes two years to complete its life cycle. During the first year, its leaves, stems and roots grow, then it enters a period of dormancy in the winter months. Next, the plant flowers and produces fruits and seeds before it dies.

Parsley can be used to make soups, salads, and sauces in addition to being a garnish. It is often used in detoxing juice cleanses and medicinally to reduce the risk of developing certain cancers, improve the function of the immune system, reduce inflammation, protect the blood vessels, and reduce the risk of developing diseases such as type 2 diabetes and asthma.

To plant parsley, individual seeds need to be placed in pots indoors for 10 to 12 weeks before the last spring frost. Soaking the seeds overnight before planting makes for better germination. The seeds should be planted in moist, rich soil with six to eight inches between them. The soil should be around 70 degrees Fahrenheit for best growth. Placing a fluorescent light above the seedlings makes them grow faster and healthier. When planting parsley, it is best to place them near tomatoes, corn, and asparagus in your garden. Continue to water the seeds daily so that they do not dry out during the process of germination.

Parsley is ready to be harvested when the leaf stems have three segments. The leaves from the outer portions can be cut, but the inner portions should be left on the plant to mature. Parsley can be stored by placing the stalk in water and keeping refrigerated or in dry storage by cutting the base of the parsley and hanging them in a well-ventilated warm and shady area. Once the parsley has completely dried, crumble it and store in an airtight container. You can enjoy parsley throughout the winter by replanting the parsley plant in a container and keeping it near a sunny window indoors.

## *Thyme*

This herb is used to make soups, grilled meat, and vegetables taste wonderful. It is a fragrant herb that has small leaves and a thin wooden stem. It comes in over 50 varieties and originated from the Mediterranean. Its health benefits include lowering blood pressure, boosting immunity, being a cough suppressant, being an insect repellent and a mood booster.

Thyme is an herb that loves heat and grows best in temperatures of around 70 degrees Fahrenheit. The soil needs to be well-drained. It is easiest to grow thyme from the plant cuttings around two to three weeks before the last spring frost. Plant the cuttings about nine inches apart. Thyme should be grown next to tomatoes and cabbages in your garden. Just like rosemary, this can be transplanted to a container in the winter months and left next to a sunny window to grow.

This plant should be watered deeply only when the soil has completely dried out. It should be pruned in the spring and summer months to contain its growth. This plant needs to be replaced when they are about three to four years old because the leaves become less flavorful and the stem becomes woodier.

Thyme can be harvested by cutting about five inches of growth while leaving the lower your parts behind. It is best to harvest thyme in the morning before the dew has dried out. Thyme should be stored and refrigerated for one to two weeks while lightly packaged in plastic. For drying thyme, hang the sprigs in a well-ventilated, warm and dry area. When the spring have dried out, crush them and store in an airtight container for up to two years.

### *Mint*

This herb has a fruity aromatic taste and flowers pink, purple, and white buds. This plant has several varieties. This plant spreads very easily so you need to be careful where you plant it. Mint thrives in well-drained soil and may require some protection from direct sunlight. When mint is grown indoors, it is best to grow it in a confined area such as a container, especially since they needed protection in the colder months of winter. Plant mint next to tomatoes and cabbages in a garden.

Mint is propagated by using cuttings that are about six inches long. These need to be placed horizontally in the soil or placed to root in a glass of water.

Mint does not require much care. When it is planted outdoors, use light mulch to keep the soil moist and the leaves clean. When it is planted indoors, it needs to be watered regularly to keep the soil moist.

Mint needs to be harvested frequently due to its penchant for overgrowth and because young leaves have more flavor than older ones. Mint can be harvested as soon as it pops up in spring. Mint can be stored frozen or air-dried.

## Basil

Basil is great for bring flavor to soups, smoothies, juices, Italian dishes, pesto, and as a garnish. This plant thrives in warm weather. The most common types of basil are sweet basil, purple basil, lemon basil, and Thai basil. Even though basil is easy to grow and maintain, it should only be grown outdoors in summer. Ideally, it should be planted six weeks before the last spring frost and after the well-drained but moist soil has warmed up to at least 70 degrees Fahrenheit. Nighttime temperature should not go below 50 degrees Fahrenheit. The plant also needs to be planted in an area that gets between six and eight hours of sunlight daily. Without this heat, the plant will not grow.

To plant basil, the seeds should be placed about ¼-inch deep into the soil with about 12 inches placed between. Basil grow best when planted next to tomatoes.

After the bud has produced at least six leaves, prune the plant to about the second set to encourage branching. This encourages the growth of more leaves for harvesting. Repeat this pruning process every time that the basil produced their first set of leaves. Pinch off the center six-weeks after germination to prevent early flowering. If flowers grow, cut them off.

If the weather suddenly becomes cold, harvest the plant because the chilly weather will destroy it.

## *Winter Savory*

The scientific name of winter savory is satureja montana. It is an annual plant and has a strong, peppery flavor. The plant has dark green, glossy leaves, and woody stems. It grows best when exposed to at least six hours of sunlight daily and when planted in well-drained soil that has a pH of 6.7. The seeds should be planted in spring outdoors in pots and transplanted to a garden about 10 inches apart. Winter savory can also be propagated through cuttings in late spring. The cuttings should be placed in pots filled with wet sand. The sprouts can then be transplanted to a container or garden. This plant will become dormant in the winter months and will put out new leaves in spring. Pruning encourages new growth. The health benefits of this plant include treating diarrhea and nausea, treating sore throats, as a tonic, as a cough suppressant and to increase sex drive.

This planted can be used to make essential oils. The leaves can also be used fresh or dried.

## *Oregano*

This plant can be used to fight bacterial infections, for its anti-cancer properties, for its antioxidant properties, to reduce viral infections, and to decrease inflammation. This herb has a taste that is similar to thyme and can be used in a variety of tasty dishes. It is commonly used in Italian dishes.

This is a plant that loves warm weather, and it is usually planted late in the spring season. It can be propagated from seeds or cuttings between 6 and 10 weeks before the last spring frost. Either seeds or cuttings can be placed in well-drained soil that has a temperature of around 70 degrees Fahrenheit. Plants should be planted at least 10 inches apart and can be planted next to any vegetable or herb in your garden.

To care for oregano plants, allow them to grow to about four-inches tall and then trim to encourage branching and higher leaf density. Oregano is a plant that does not require much care and does not need to be watered as often as most herbs. Water the oregano when the soil feels dry.

Leaves can be harvested as needed and the most flavorful ones are found right before the plant blooms flowers. Oregon leaves can be stored by freezing and air drying them. Once they are dried, keep them stored in an airtight container.

## *Sage*

Sage, whose scientific name is salvia officinalis, is a plant that is easy to grow and adds a lot of flavor to dishes, especially meats and bean dishes. The leaves of the sage plant are gray-green in color and its flowers can be blue, pink, white, and purple.

Sage will not grow in wet soil; therefore, should be planted in well-drained soil. The best and easiest way to propagate sage is from a small plant. Seeds can also be planted two weeks before the last spring frost. Cuttings can be planted one or two weeks before the last spring frost.

Soil temperature should be between 60 and 70 degrees Fahrenheit, and plants should be grown in close proximity to rosemary, cabbage and carrots in a garden. Keep them far away from cucumbers.

To care for sage, the young plants should be watered regularly so that they grow quickly at which point watering can be decreased. It is best to replace these plants every few years. They should be pruned every spring.

To harvest sage, harvest lightly during the first year of growth by pinching off the leaves or by snipping off small sprigs from the plant. Once the first year has passed, you only need to leave a few stalks so that the plants can rejuvenate in the future. Once the plant has fully established itself, it can be harvested up to three times in one season. Do not harvest the plant in the fall so that it can prepare for winter. Sage can be stored by freezing or drying, it but can be used fresh as well.

The health benefits of sage include being an antioxidant, supporting good oral health, easing the symptoms of menopause, reducing blood sugar levels, supporting brain health, lowering bad cholesterol levels, protecting against certain cancers, alleviating diarrhea and supporting bone health.

## *Sorrel*

Sorel is an herb with a tangy, lemony flavor. The flowers are commonly used to make juices. The sorrel leaves can be steamed or sautéed just as you would spinach. They can also be used in salads, soups, and sauces. The leaves are commonly used in French cuisine. There are several varieties of sorrel, but they are all known for the health benefits of lowering blood pressure, decreasing bad cholesterol levels, detoxifying the body and as an antioxidant.

Sorrel grows in temperate conditions in damp soil in open areas. Sorrel can be sown from the seeds or by dividing the roots. The best time to propagate sorrel is in June or July. The flowers bloom quickly after and can be used to make juice. This slows down the production of leaves so if you want more leaf production, cut off the flower stalks. Cutting off the flower stalks also gives you more harvests. You can cut the plant to the ground and it will produce a new crop.

Sorrel can be harvested late in the spring until fall or when the plant is about six inches tall. Both the flower and the leaves can be harvested.

# Conclusion

Billions of dollars are exchanged every year for the human race to obtain healthcare. Every year the amount spent increases because every year pharmaceutical companies find new ways of ensuring we are tricked into thinking that they are dependent on prescription drugs to make living bearable. We have been duped into believing that life cannot no longer be a fun, enjoyable, healthy adventure because sickness is spreading like wildfire and this is all part of the propaganda designed by these big name companies.

It is a sad truth that human disease and illness is a big business for the pharmaceutical companies and doctors. These are the people we have placed our faith in to keep us healthy but that trust is being broken because pharmaceutical drugs come with a host of side effects that can make us even more unwell than when they started the use of pharmaceutical drugs. Even more unfortunate is the fact that these side effects are considered mild most times. How can they possibly be mild when they disrupt our daily lives and lower the quality of the way we live? How can being a diarrhea or suffering from dizziness or nausea be considered mild when you cannot leave the house for fear that these side effects will embarrass you or place your life in danger?

And what of the more 'serious' side effects like internal bleeding, liver damage, and heart disease that are whispered in commercials like the inconsequential? But these side effects are far from inconsequential. They matter just as your health and wellness does. And it is an insult us that pharmaceutical downplay the severity of these side effects.

It is time that we stopped being slaves to pharmaceutical companies and doctors that use our pain for their gain. There is a better way to obtain the good health that you desire, and it comes free of charge most often. Human health is the most valuable resource that we will ever own and it is about time that it be treated with the high worth that it has.

## Plant-Based Medicine Worked for Our Ancestors and It Can Work for You Too

Before the invention of technology and money, our ancestors took to the earth and planted herbs and spices that they used to treat illnesses that range from mild to serious. There was no monopoly of resources or manipulation for profit. Our ancestors simply when outside and pick a plant from the garden to find a cure for an illness and to prevent the development of a disease. This seems like a lost time, but it does not have to be. You too can benefit from naturally grown medications instead of risking your health with synthetics.

## Plant-Based Eating Can Change Your Life for the Better

Plants not only provide us with powerful medicinal effects but they also provide us with powerful nutrition, detoxification, and other health benefits such as improved function of the immune system and lowered risk of developing several other diseases such as obesity, cardiovascular disease, digestive issues, and mental illness. The powerful compounds in plants are so effective that pharmaceutical companies try to imitate the effects. But nothing beats the natural way.

## Take Control of Your Overall Health

The pages of this book are packed with powerful information that allows you to take control of not only your health but your entire life because they not only contain information on medicinal practices but how to improve your eating habits and detoxify your body. There is nothing stopping you from being the healthier, happier, and more productive individual that you can be. It is possible to cure and prevent illnesses without suffering from side effects. It is possible to eat healthier without having to drive through a restaurant that serves questionable ingredients and buy ingredients that are filled with the remnants of fertilizers. It is possible to get rid of the toxins that modern pollution and bad eating habits have made common in the human body. It is possible to make your immune system stronger than ever by fortifying it with nutrition and probiotics.

All of this and more are possible by stepping out into your yard or plucking a leaf from your kitchen garden. You can control your health to such an extent that you do not even have to go to the grocery store to stock up on healthy eating and medicinal ingredients. You can get it all right there in your own garden even if you live in a small space.

## *A Final Word*

We all want to live healthier lives. Being in good health makes us happier, less stressed, and makes life feel like it is worth living. Being sick can drain us and make life seem hopeless, especially when you have been prescribed pill after pill and tablet upon tablet and you are seeing little to no results. This kind of life is no better than living as a slave and, in this case, it is being a slave to pharmaceutical corporations that bank on you never fully recovering. Fortunately, you can break free of the shackles at any time on any day. Taking a plant-based approach to medicine and diet places you as the one in control of your life, which is the way that it should.

This book was written with careful consideration and packed with tons of knowledge to place you well on your way to living a life that is healthier and therefore, happier. I hope that the tips outlined have been solidified in your mind so that you can start acting today. None of these tips will do any good if you do not get proactive. You need to take action to see the results. If you need to, do not be afraid to go back and read the particular sections that are of interest to you. While you are at it, share this book with a friend or family member so that they too can break free of the shackles that pharmaceutical companies have imprisoned us with.

# References

Bent S. (2008). Herbal medicine in the United States: a review of efficacy, safety, and regulation: grand rounds at the University of California, San Francisco Medical Center. *Journal of general internal medicine, 23*(6), 854–859. doi:10.1007/s11606-008-0632-y

DeAngelis C. D. (2016). Big Pharma Profits and the Public Loses. *The Milbank quarterly, 94*(1), 30–33. doi:10.1111/1468-0009.12171

Ferner R. E. (2005). The influence of big pharma. *BMJ (Clinical research ed.), 330*(7496), 855–856. doi:10.1136/bmj.330.7496.855

Firenzuoli, F., & Gori, L. (2007). Herbal medicine today: clinical and research issues. *Evidence-based complementary and alternative medicine : eCAM, 4*(Suppl 1), 37–40. doi:10.1093/ecam/nem096

Hajar R. (2012). The air of history: early medicine to galen (part I). *Heart views : the official journal of the Gulf Heart Association, 13*(3), 120–128. doi:10.4103/1995-705X.102164

Nicholson L. B. (2016). The immune system. *Essays in biochemistry, 60*(3), 275–301. doi:10.1042/EBC20160017

Ostfeld R. J. (2017). Definition of a plant-based diet and overview of this special issue. *Journal of geriatric cardiology : JGC, 14*(5), 315. doi:10.11909/j.issn.1671-5411.2017.05.008

Rang H. (2013). Bad Pharma: how drug companies mislead doctors and harm patients. *British Journal of Clinical Pharmacology, 75*(5), 1377–1379. doi:10.1111/bcp.12047

Welz, A. N., Emberger-Klein, A., & Menrad, K. (2018). Why people use herbal medicine: insights from a focus-group study in Germany. *BMC complementary and alternative medicine, 18*(1), 92. doi:10.1186/s12906-018-2160-6